Competence Training for Pharmacy

Special Issue Editor
Jeffrey Atkinson

MDPI • Basel • Beijing • Wuhan • Barcelona • Belgrade

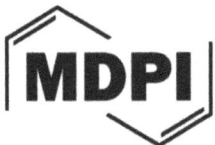

MDPI

Special Issue Editor
Jeffrey Atkinson
Pharmacolor Consultants Nancy
France

Editorial Office
MDPI AG
St. Alban-Anlage 66
Basel, Switzerland

This edition is a reprint of the Special Issue published online in the open access journal *Pharmacy* (ISSN 2226-4787) in 2017 (available at: http://www.mdpi.com/journal/pharmacy/special_issues/competence_training).

For citation purposes, cite each article independently as indicated on the article page online and as indicated below:

Author 1; Author 2. Article title. *Journal Name* **Year**, *Article number*, page range.

First Edition 2017

ISBN 978-3-03842-480-2 (Pbk)
ISBN 978-3-03842-481-9 (PDF)

Photo courtesy of PCN, Villers, France

Table of Contents

About the Special Issue Editor

Jeffrey Atkinson, Emeritus professor, Lorraine University, France. Jeffrey Atkinson followed an initial career in cardiovascular pharmacology and physiology in the UK, USA, Italy, Switzerland and France. In parallel, he taught cardiovascular pharmacology and therapy in the Faculty of Medicine of Lausanne University, and the Faculty of Pharmacy of Lorraine University, France. For the past 15 years, his interests have centred more on pharmacy education and training with a special interest in the development of new methods. He has directed several European programmes aimed at harmonising pharmacy education and training in Europe, and developing a European model for pharmacy education and training based on competence training.

Preface to "Competence Training for Pharmacy"

The pharmacy community is showing a growing interest in competence-based education (CBE) as a shift is seen in many countries, away from education structured by resources, curricula and time-frames. CBE is more easily understood by society and provides a clearer public statement of the role of the pharmacist. Furthermore, CBE can help in the mutual recognition of qualifications promoting student and practitioner mobility. Finally, the CBE approach can also facilitate the development of advanced, specialized practice.

This book brings together distinguished, international specialists who describe the various facets of CBE from philosophy and implications to methodology and development, and finally to application and experience.

In the first chapter of the book, Melissa Medina from the University of Oklahoma, USA, reviews the evolution of pharmacy education in the USA and offers insight into the benefits and challenges of the future use of CBE in pharmacy education in the USA. Based on experience of teaching pharmacy, Ieva Stupans from the RMIT University in Victoria, Australia, reviews the literature around competence outcomes regarding students' communication skills and the development of accountability, proposing a model to guide the selection of teaching and assessment approaches for accountability. Andries Koster and colleagues from the University of Utrecht, The Netherlands, propose a detailed iterative process for the implementation of CBE. John Hawboldt and colleagues from Memorial University, St. John's, Canada and the University of Tasmania, Australia, consider international exchanges between Canada and Australia and the alignment of local standards with the Global Competency Framework of the International Pharmaceutical Federation. This approach may facilitate greater international mobility in the future. Rose Nash and colleagues from the Universities of Tasmania, Queensland, Brisbane, and Victoria, Australia, examine how competence training for pharmacists may enhance the quality of continued professional development (CPD). They argue that the competence required to engage in meaningful CPD practice should be introduced and developed prior to entry into practice.

The second part of the book deals with the European experience. Howard Davies from the European University Association in Brussels, Belgium, describes the twin-track nature of the organisation of European higher education with the intergovernmental action programme of the Bologna Process running alongside the developments in EU legislation. Taking as an example the sectoral profession of pharmacy, he shows how the development of CBE could bring the two policy tracks into closer alignment. Antonio Sanchez-Pozo from the University of Granada, Spain, compares competences for pharmacy practice in Europe with those for medicine and dentistry. He shows that the rankings of the vast majority of competences for medicine and pharmacy are remarkably similar. This result lays the foundation for the design of more interdisciplinary educational programs for healthcare professionals based on CBE, and for the development of team-based care. The European PHAR-QA (Quality Assurance in European Pharmacy Education and Training) consortium then describes the production of the European Pharmacy Competence Framework (EPCF). In two subsiduary chapters, Constantin Mircioiu from the "Carol Davila" University of Medicine and Pharmacy, Bucharest, Romania and Jeffrey Atkinson, from the University of Lorraine, France, elaborate further on methodological aspects of the production of the EPCF, especially those concerning the statistical approaches to the ranking of competences by the pharmacy community. The final four chapters deal with the mapping of existing curricula to the EPCF and the possibilities for the development of the latter at the Universities of: Helsinki, Finland (Nina Katajavuori and colleagues), Tartu, Estonia (Daisy Volmer and colleagues), Ljubljana, Slovenia (Tanja Gmeiner and colleagues), and Krakow, Poland (Agnieszka Skowron and colleagues). These chapters illustrate how the EPCF can be used as a tool for reflection and optimization of pharmacy curricula in different local contexts.

Jeffrey Atkinson
Special Issue Editor

pharmacy

MDPI

Review

Does Competency-Based Education Have a Role in Academic Pharmacy in the United States?

Melissa S. Medina

College of Pharmacy, The University of Oklahoma, 1110 N Stonewall Ave, Oklahoma City, OK 73117, USA;
Melissa-medina@ouhsc.edu; Tel.: +1-405-271-6484

Academic Editor: Jeffrey Atkinson
Received: 20 January 2017; Accepted: 20 February 2017; Published: 27 February 2017

Abstract: Competency-based Education (CBE) is an educational model that allows students to learn and demonstrate their abilities at their own pace. CBE is growing in popularity in undergraduate educational programs and its role in pharmacy education in the United States (US) is under review. In comparison, medical education is utilizing competency-based approaches (such as competencies and Entrustable Professional Activities) to ensure that students possess the required knowledge, skills, and attitudes prior to graduation or program completion. The concept of competency-based approaches is growing in use in pharmacy education in the US, but the future related to aspects of this concept (e.g., mandatory Entrustable Professional Activities) is not certain. A review of pharmacy education's evolution in the US and a comparison of competency-related terms offers insight into the future use of competency-based approaches and CBE in pharmacy education in the US through the lens of benefits and challenges.

Keywords: competence; pharmacy; healthcare; program outcomes; education; standards

1. Introduction

In the United States (US), medical education has increased its interest in Competency-based Education (CBE) over the past several years, which has piqued interest in pharmacy. Formally, a CBE program is an educational model that removes traditional semester timeframes, allowing students to learn at their own pace and demonstrate what they know through assessments developed by the program [1]. Relatedly, competency-based approaches (including assessment of competencies) have been used in educational programs such as pharmacy, as seen in the 2016 Accreditation Council for Pharmacy Education (ACPE) Standards program outcomes which use the term competencies in relationship to outcomes [2,3]. It is important to note that a competency-based approach and competencies in pharmacy education are different than formal CBE, which removes semester timeframes. In order to understand the future of CBE in pharmacy education in the US, it is important to reflect on the past and present of pharmacy education; define the terminology related to CBE and competencies, and evaluate how other health professions (such as medical education) address CBE and competencies, which can offer insight into future directions for pharmacy education.

2. History of Pharmacy Education Standards

In the US in the 19th century, there was no legal requirement to learn the pharmacy profession through formal education and the apprenticeship model was the dominant training method [4]. State universities were the first to design formal pharmacist education models, starting in 1868 at the University of Michigan, where students enrolled in full-day courses over four terms (3-months long each) and no prior pharmacy work experience was required for admittance and in 1892, the University of Wisconsin established a four-year program [4]. During the 20th and 21st centuries, the Flexner report precipitated changes to the content and length of the pharmacy curriculum, mode of delivery, required prerequisites, and the degree earned [4,5]. There was also little uniformity in pharmacy licensure and no program accrediting bodies until 1932 when ACPE was founded [4].

The US Department of Education (USDE) now recognizes ACPE as the organization that evaluates the quality of professional degree programs leading to the Doctor of Pharmacy degree, the standard entry level degree. To receive accreditation, Doctor of Pharmacy programs must meet expectations outlined in the 2016 ACPE Accreditation standards [2]. During the 20th and 21st centuries ACPE has overseen many changes in pharmacy education such as the length of the program from 4 to 6 years and the entry level degree from Bachelor of Science to Doctor of Pharmacy. Recently, major changes have occurred regarding how programs are delivered and there are now accelerated 3-year programs, online programs, and multi-site campuses that are connected through synchronous video-streaming. These changes to program delivery have resulted in changes to the accreditation standards, with the most recent update occurring in 2016 [2]. The reverse is also true, where changes in the accreditation standards have required changes to pharmacy curricula. The 2016 ACPE standards include emphasis on an affective domain (standard 4) based on the 2013 CAPE outcomes revision [2]. The growing importance of interprofessional education is seen in standard 11 [2] and the administration of the Pharmacy Curriculum Outcomes Assessment (PCOA) in the pre-advanced pharmacy practice experience (Pre-APPE) is delineated in standard 12 [2]. Standard 10 outlines Curriculum Design, Deliver, and Oversight requirements and states that the minimum curriculum duration is a minimum of four years of full–time study or the equivalent [2,6]. Standard 10.3 (knowledge application) and Standard 10.4 (skill development) indicate that students must demonstrate their competencies in both knowledge and skills and as a result, assessment of these competencies has grown in importance [2]. These significant events are outlined in Figure 1.

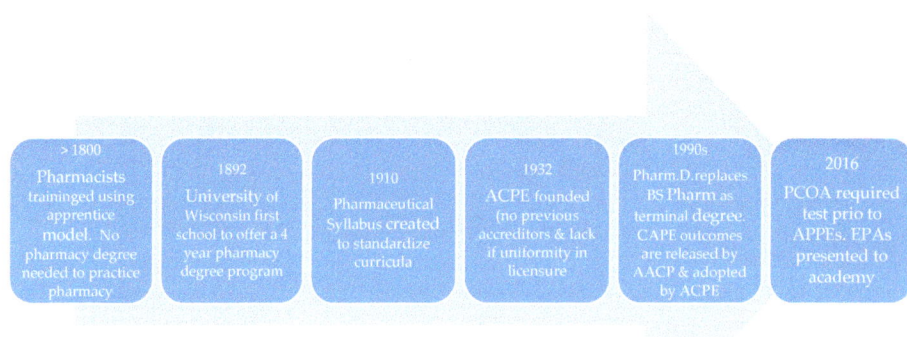

Figure 1. Timeline of Significant Pharmacy Curriculum Events in the US. ACPE = Accreditation Council for Pharmacy Education. AACP = American Association of Colleges of Pharmacy. CAPE = Center for the Advancement of Pharmacy Education outcomes; which are revised every 7 years (current version is 2013). PCOA = Pharmacy Curriculum Outcomes Assessment. APPE = Advanced Pharmacy Practice Experiences. EPA = Entrustable Professional Activities.

3. Definitions of Competency-Based Education (CBE) and Competency-Based Approaches

The growing importance of assessment has increased the terminology and concepts related to assessment. One of these newer concepts that has arisen in higher education is the term competency-based education. Higher education has historically used time (e.g., semesters and credit hours-formally known as the Carnegie Unit) as the yardstick for determining readiness, which arose in the early 1900s and formed the basis for program design, accreditation, and funding [1,7]. CBE in contrast emphasizes directly measuring how much students have learned (learning-based system) instead of how long they have spent learning (time–based system), which allows students to move at their own pace [1]. CBE programs are aimed at nontraditional students who need more flexible options to earn their first or second degree or update their skills [1]. These programs are more than just on-line programs because the focus instead turns to allowing students to demonstrate their achievement of required competencies which may have been gained during previous work experience, therefore allowing the more flexible awarding of credit in comparison to credit hours [7]. In CBE, students demonstrate mastery of explicit and measurable knowledge, skill, and attitude outcomes (competencies) and receive individualized support that is tailored to their specific developmental needs [7]. Students progress in the program by demonstrating they have mastered the knowledge and skills (competencies) for a course regardless of time, meaning they could take more or less time [8], therefore studying and learning at their own pace. CBE allows students to accelerate through what they already know and spend more time on what they do not know, which means students can accelerate (or delay) their progress toward a degree [8]. A comparison of traditional versus CBE can be seen in Table 1.

Table 1. Comparison of traditional vs. competency based education.

Curricular Concept	Traditional Instruction	CBE
Structure	Time-based, semesters and credit hours	Learner-centered; Competency-based
Teaching mode	Group learning, emphasis on knowledge	Individualized, tailored, emphasis on abilities or competencies
Pace	Faculty-paced; all students move together through content at same time; structured	Self-paced; movement through content determined by individual student's competency attainment; flexible
Assessment method	Summative, high stakes	Mastery-learning, performance-based
Program completion time	Finish when all required courses are passed	Finish when mastery of competencies demonstrated

In comparison to CBE, which focuses on changing the structure and time requirements of educational programs, ultimately changing curricula, there are competency-based approaches that embed the teaching of competencies and assessment of competence into the existing curricula and traditional time-based structure [3]. Competency-based approaches are currently used in undergraduate and medical education and their use is growing in pharmacy education [3,9,10]. Therefore, the future of competency-based approaches is now. Within this approach, there are competencies, which are predefined abilities or outcomes of a curriculum [10]. There is also competence that can be thought of as progression toward professional expertise or demonstration of a predefined skill or knowledge level that is multi-dimensional, dynamic, contextual, and developmental [10]. Competencies describe qualities of professionals and measuring professional competence can be difficult [11]. One way that medicine has evaluated competencies of their students or trainees within the medical curricula is to use Entrustable Professional Activities (EPAs) [12] and pharmacy education has focused recent attention on EPAs as well [3]. The terms EPA and competencies should not be used interchangeably because EPAs are descriptors of work and translate competencies in professional practice whereas competencies describe physicians [11,12]. Outlining core EPAs is a way to ensure that students are practice ready upon graduation [3] which is an aim of the 2016 ACPE Accreditation Standards [2]. EPAs reflect the level of supervision required for students (e.g., direct vs. distant supervision) and are aimed at establishing the level of proficiency that is required for professional practice upon completion of training or graduation [11]. When an EPA is first learned and practiced, the level of supervision needed may be high, which would be considered developmentally appropriate and expected for early leaners [3,11].

Competency-based approaches as described above are currently in use and development. In the future, although the EPAs are not officially required in the ACPE standards 2016, it is possible they will follow the path of the CAPE Outcomes and become adopted in the standards [2,6]. It is also possible that in the future, EPAs may set the stage for required mandatory skills-based examinations (such as Objective Structured Clinical Exams), similar to the PCOA exam The ACPE standards 2016 have become more prescriptive in this version related to assessment as a way for programs to increase their transparency while working on continuous quality improvement [2]. Key elements in Section 3 require formative and summative assessments as well as mandatory, standardized, and comparative assessments [2]. This section also discusses student achievement and readiness to "enter APPE, provide direct patient care in a variety of settings, and contribute to an Interprofessional collaborative patient care team" [2] (p. 25). The assessment standards offer colleges and schools of pharmacy more guidance on how they should demonstrate that their students have learned and achieved the educational outcomes and as a result, an OSCE-like exam based on competencies and EPAs is possible.

While competency-based approaches are emerging in current pharmacy curricula with attention on EPAs, the appeal is that the competency based assessment can provide a mechanism to prevent students from graduating from a pharmacy program unless they have demonstrated the predefined and expected level of competence for program outcomes [3]. This appeal is a subtle yet important distinction because in its current and near future use EPAs require students to demonstrate and achieve OR remediate deficient knowledge and skills prior to graduation within the existing curricular structure. Students can take more time if needed but it must be completed within the allotted timeframe and academic standing policies. EPAs do not currently allow an open-ended and limitless timeframe. Although competency-based approaches are used in medicine and pharmacy, it is unclear what the future holds for formal CBE. There are benefits and challenges to the design.

4. Benefits and Challenges of CBE in Pharmacy Education

Frank and colleagues [10] described benefits to medical education and these benefits can be extrapolated to pharmacy education. (1) Defines consistent competencies and milestones. CBE would help pharmacy educators define competencies expected of graduates and developmental milestones prior to graduation, better ensuring that all students possess the same level of baseline skills upon graduation; (2) Determines acceptable levels of performance for competencies and milestones. CBE would promote a national discussion of what constitutes an acceptable level of evidence of abilities; such as when are students expected to demonstrate novice, competent, proficient, or expert performance for specific competencies. This would better align faculty expectations so that one faculty member does not expect a higher or lower level than another faculty member; (3) Outlines acceptable assessment methods and tools for assessing the competencies. CBE would shape what assessments best measure the outcomes of specific competencies. It would also better ensure that assessment of graduates' abilities would not vary as a result of programmatic, regional, or local differences; (4) Offers flexibility in learning. CBE would offer students a more flexible timeframe to demonstrate competencies and therefore allow them to progress at their own rate, which is more learner centered and personalized [10].

There are challenges associated with CBE in pharmacy education which can be inferred from medicine [10]. (1) Presents IPPE and APPE logistical concerns. The biggest challenge to using CBE is that moving students through time-based curricula is efficient and manageable. For example, it is unclear how programs will accommodate students on introductory and advanced pharmacy practice experiences (IPPE and APPE) when the prescribed number of weeks is removed but preceptor laws remain and some sites can only accommodate a limited number of students; (2) Complicates faculty time allocation. When students complete course content at different times, it is unclear how faculty would handle assessment of knowledge, skills, and attitudes in an efficient manner. There is an efficiency to administering exams to an entire class during a set time block. It is possible that faculty would spend a majority of their time assessing knowledge, skills, and attitudes on an individual basis for the didactic portion of the program, leaving little time to teach and assess on IPPE and APPEs as well as fulfill other parts of the tripartite mission; (3) Makes managing poor student performance and progression difficult. Pharmacy curricula are designed to have courses and content build upon each other. While students can self-pace, much of the course work is lock-step in nature. It is not clear how programs will manage students completing prescriptive course work at different rates. In addition, many programs have some rate of attrition due to poor performance. Academic standing committees would need to establish time limits and maximum number of attempts for students to complete competencies, which could be logistically difficult to manage. CBE is also less structured by design, which may lead to more student dismissals as a result of weak students who may not manage their time well. The structure offered in time-based curricula can benefit academically at-risk students, whereas the lack of structure in CBE may hurt that category of students; (4) Creates a narrow focus of curricula. A focus on completing competencies can shift attention from the big picture of how content within a curriculum builds up and advances to a more fragmented picture of small units of performance and "jumping through hoops" which can frustrate faculty and students [10]. Focus can also shift from learning goals to performance goals, which are indicative of a fixed mindset where students are more likely to cheat, give up when faced with failure, and focus on receiving validation from others instead of striving for competence and mastery [13,14]; (5) Shifts attention from knowledge to skills. Previous complaints have arisen that pharmacy is too content heavy and that students may enter professional practice lacking skills. Shifting to CBE may create an imbalance in the opposite direction where skills are more valued than knowledge, emphasizing the role of the pharmacist as a technician versus a health-care provider and problem-solver.

5. Discussion

Overall, CBE is an instructional model that is built on eliminating time-based curricula. Based on this definition, the use of CBE in US pharmacy education is unclear. A review of the literature suggests the CBE definition is applied broadly and the future of the concept competency-based approaches (e.g., EPAs) where attention is placed on students demonstrating competencies during the traditional time-limited and structured program is currently being implemented and grown in pharmacy education. There are still areas of future uncertainty related to competency-based approaches such as mandatory EPAs and required national OSCE assessments in ACPE program accreditation. The future of formal CBE in pharmacy education has benefits and challenges. CBE appears to be difficult to implement, especially in a political climate where colleges and universities are asked to do more with less money and resources. While the pharmacy academy may benefit from ensuring that students can meet specific competencies at predefined levels along the expert-novice continuum, removing time-based curricula may not be feasible in the immediate future.

Conflicts of Interest: The authors declare no conflict of interest.

References

1. Kamenetz, A. NPR-Education, Higher Education: Competency-Based Education: No More Semesters? Available online: http://www.npr.org/sections/ed/2014/10/07/353930358/competency-based-education-no-more-semesters (accessed on 13 December 2016).
2. Accreditation Council for Pharmacy Education. Accreditation Standards and Key Elements for the Professional Program in Pharmacy Leading to the Doctor of Pharmacy Degree, 2015. Available online: https://www.acpe-accredit.org/standards/ (accessed on 13 December 2016).
3. Pittenger, A.L.; Chapman, S.A.; Frail, C.K.; Chapman, S.A.; Moon, J.Y.; Undeberg, M.R.; Orzoff, J.H. Entrustable professional activities for pharmacy practice. *Am. J. Pharm. Educ.* **2016**, *80*, 57. [CrossRef] [PubMed]
4. Mrtek, R.G. Contemporary pharmaceutical education in these United States-An interpretive historical essay of the twentieth century. *Am. J. Pharm. Educ.* **1976**, *40*, 339–365. [PubMed]
5. Flexner, A. *Medical Education in the United States and Canada: A Report to the Carnegie Foundation for the Advancement of Teaching*; Carnegie Foundation for the Advancement of Teaching: New York, NY, USA, 1910.

6. Medina, M.S.; Plaza, C.M.; Stowe, C.D.; Robinson, E.T.; DeLander, G.; Beck, D.E.; Melchert, R.B.; Supernaw, R.B.; Roche, V.F.; Gleason, B.L.; et al. Center for the Advancement of Pharmacy Education (CAPE) 2013 educational outcomes. *Am. J. Pharm. Educ.* **2013**, *77*, 162. [CrossRef] [PubMed]
7. Competency Works: Learning from the Cutting Edge. Available online: http://www.competencyworks. org/about/competency-education/ (accessed on 13 December 2016).
8. Mendenhall, R. What Is Competency-Based Education? 2012, Huffington Post. Available online: http://www.huffingtonpost.com/dr-robert-mendenhall/competency-based-learning-_b_1855374.html (accessed on 13 December 2016).
9. Fain, P. Competency-Based Education Arrives at Three Major Public Institutions. Inside Higher Ed. Available online: https://www.insidehighered.com/news/2014/10/28/competency-based-education-arrives-three-major-public-institutions (accessed on 13 December 2016).
10. Frank, J.R.; Snell, L.S.; Cate, O.T.; Holmboe, E.S.; Carraccio, C.; Swing, S.R.; Harris, P.; Glasgow, N.J.; Campbell, C.; et al. Competency-based medical education: Theory to practice. *Med. Teach.* **2010**, *32*, 638–645. [CrossRef] [PubMed]
11. Ten Cate O. Nuts and bolts of entrustable professional activities. *J. Grad. Med. Educ.* **2013**, *5*, 157–158. [CrossRef] [PubMed]
12. Ten Cate O. Entrustability of professional activities and competency-based training. *Med. Educ.* **2005**, *39*, 1176–1177. [CrossRef] [PubMed]
13. Dweck, C.S. Can personality be changed? The role of beliefs in personality and change. *Curr. Direct. Psychol. Sci.* **2008**, *17*, 391–394. [CrossRef]
14. Murphy, M.C.; Dweck, C.S. A culture of genius: How an organization's lay theories shape people's cognition, affect, and behavior. *Personal. Soc. Psychol. Bull.* **2010**, *36*, 283–296. [CrossRef] [PubMed]

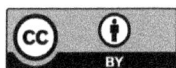

pharmacy

MDPI

Article

A Curriculum Challenge—The Need for Outcome (Competence) Descriptors

Ieva Stupans

School of Health and Biomedical Sciences, RMIT University, PO Box 71 Bundoora, Victoria 3083, Australia; ieva.stupans@rmit.edu.au

Academic Editor: Jeffrey Atkinson
Received: 16 November 2016; Accepted: 10 February 2017; Published: 17 February 2017

Abstract: Some outcomes around, for example, communication have been extensively theorised; others such as accountability have been relatively neglected in the teaching and learning literature. The question therefore is: if we do not have a clear understanding of the outcome, can we systematically apply good practice principles in course design such that students are able to achieve the outcomes the community and the profession expect? This paper compares and contrasts the literature around competency outcomes regarding students' communication skills and the development of accountability and proposes a model to guide the selection of teaching and assessment approaches for accountability, based on the students' sphere of influence.

Keywords: accountability; communication; competencies; learning outcomes

1. Introduction

Our ability as educators to evaluate the effectiveness of our teaching depends, in part, on our ability to assess students' learning. One of the key principles of good practice in curriculum design and in teaching is that of alignment between outcomes, learning opportunities and assessment. Suitable assessments can be designed only once standards for attainment have been clearly identified. The Competency Outcomes and Performance Assessment Model (COPA) provides a simple framework for competency-based or outcomes-based education. These are: (1) What are the essential competencies and outcomes for contemporary practice? (2) What are the indicators that define those competencies? (3) What are the most effective ways to learn those competencies? (4) What are the most effective ways to document that learners have achieved the required competencies [1]? The questions within this framework essentially capture the constructively aligned curriculum paradigm in which the desired learning outcomes are expressed in terms of activities students are required to be able to demonstrate, with teaching and learning activities and assessment being designed to be consistent with these desired learning outcomes [2]. The process of defining outcomes is critical as the outcomes determine the focus of learning and assessment; however, they also communicate external reference points at the national and international levels both within and outside the profession. An improvement in students' being "able to do" allows the inference of the achievement of the desired learning outcomes and potentially the impact of our teaching.

In the health care literature, the terms competency, competencies, competence and competences are frequently used; these terms imply the ability to perform specific tasks, actions or functions successfully. The use of these terms also aligns with educational achievement by students, essentially a capacity or skill that is developed by the student. Competence is an outcome and, from the perspective of providing a program of study for students, sits within an outcome-oriented degree framework which refers to specific statements that describe what a student will be able to do in a measurable way. For the purposes of this paper the term *outcomes* will be used for both competence and learning outcome requirements. This is consistent with international standards and guidelines from the European Union [3], the United States Lumina Foundation Degree Qualifications Profile [4] and the Australian Qualifications Framework [5].

With the focus in higher education on preparing students for future employment, elements of a profession's core competencies are normally incorporated into specified outcomes (i.e., competency-based learning outcomes) for that profession's education programs. In the case of pharmacy programs, this process is well established, having been advocated in the 1997 World Health Organisation documents "The Role of the Pharmacist in the Health Care System" [6]. Anticipated end of degree outcomes for pharmacy graduates from Australia, Canada, the United Kingdom and the United States are all very similar and, with few exceptions, align well with the to the International Pharmaceutical Federation (FIP) Global Competency Framework [7]. With regard to the COPA model, essential outcomes for contemporary practice such as communication have been clearly outlined.

Learning outcomes are generally written with Bloom's taxonomy in mind—Bloom's taxonomy provides a framework for the process of learning whereby in the case of the cognitive domain, synthesis and evaluation represent the higher-order stages of thought processes. Similarly, in the affective domain, progress is demonstrated from a basic willingness to receive information for the integration of beliefs, ideas and attitudes. In the psychomotor domain, a number of taxonomies describe the development of skills and the coordination of brain and muscular activity [8]. With reference to the outcomes focused on in this paper, all three domains of Bloom's taxonomy are relevant to communication: knowledge (cognition), motivation (affect) and skills (psychomotor abilities) [9]. Communication can be enhanced or diminished by any one of these components. Development of accountability aligns with the "continuum of internalisation" of affective values [8,10]. Assessment strategies depend on the domain of learning being assessed [11]. For example, the assessment of skill levels of communication needs to be based on actual performance. As students progress through a program of study, learning outcomes may be written such that a higher level of performance is progressively expected [8]. Learning outcomes should be clearly written, be assessable and be achievable [8].

The Dreyfus model has illuminated the developmental progression around skill acquisition and knowledge articulation embedded in expert practice [12]. This developmental model describes stages from novice, advanced beginner, competent, proficient to expert [13] and can be utilised to provide a framework for student progress towards a given outcome. The Association of Faculties of Pharmacy of Canada Educational Outcomes Task Force has utilised some of the features of the model to create descriptions of outcomes at three levels—below that required to graduate, graduation level and above expected level of performance [14]. For example, students performing at a level below that required to graduate "may use their communication skills in a formulaic manner or unstructured manner, resulting in inefficient use of time and potentially ineffective intervention", whereas at a level above the expected level of performance they are able to "demonstrate an ease of communication that enables patients and other health care providers to rapidly develop trust and confidence in their professionalism and competence as a health care provider". These levels can be used as the basis for the development of specific assessment tools.

Rubrics may be used to further illustrate to students the expectations of teaching staff around learning outcomes. Rubrics provide a coherent set of criteria for assessments for the learning outcome and descriptions of levels of performance quality for these criteria [15,16]. Rubrics have the potential to promote learning by making expectations and criteria for assessments of learning outcomes explicit [17]. The Association of American Colleges and Universities has developed VALUE (Valid Assessment of Learning in Undergraduate Education) rubrics [18] for 16 learning outcomes including the development of communication skills within programs. For example, Table 1 displays two criteria, one each for written and oral communication, and for novice to proficient performance.

Table 1. Descriptors for one written and one oral communication skill (sourced directly from Association of American Colleges and Universities [18]).

Criteria	Novice to Expert Categories	Descriptor
Context of and Purpose for Writing *Includes considerations of audience, purpose, and the circumstances surrounding the writing task(s).*	Beginner: Students in the early stages	Demonstrates minimal attention to context, audience, purpose, and to the assigned tasks(s) (e.g., expectation of instructor or self as audience).
	Novice: Students in the middle stages	Demonstrates awareness of context, audience, purpose, and to the assigned tasks(s) (e.g., begins to show awareness of audience's perceptions and assumptions).
	Competent: Graduates of this course	Demonstrates adequate consideration of context, audience, and purpose and a clear focus on the assigned task(s) (e.g., the task aligns with audience, purpose, and context).
	Proficient: Graduates as new professionals	Demonstrates a thorough understanding of context, audience, and purpose that is responsive to the assigned task(s) and focuses all elements of the work
Delivery	Beginner: Students in the early stages	Delivery techniques (posture, gesture, eye contact, and vocal expressiveness) detract from the understandability of the presentation, and speaker appears uncomfortable.
	Novice: Students in the middle stages	Delivery techniques (posture, gesture, eye contact, and vocal expressiveness) make the presentation understandable, and speaker appears tentative.
	Competent: Graduates of this course	Delivery techniques (posture, gesture, eye contact, and vocal expressiveness) make the presentation interesting, and speaker appears comfortable.
	Proficient: Graduates as new professionals	Delivery techniques (posture, gesture, eye contact, and vocal expressiveness) make the presentation compelling, and speaker appears polished and confident.

2. Curriculum Design to Promote Outcomes around Communication

The COPA model requires that indicators for outcomes (competencies) are defined. A number of resources can be used to support academics in establishing standards for the attainment of outcomes concerning communication for their own university's programs. These resources include guidelines from the European Union [3], which specifies that a cycle 1 graduate (essentially equivalent to bachelor's degree) can communicate information, ideas, problems and solutions to both specialist and non-specialist audiences. The United States Lumina Foundation Degree Qualifications Profile [4] specify that at the bachelor's level, the student is able to construct sustained, coherent arguments, narratives or explications of issues, problems or technical issues and processes, in writing and at least one other medium, to general and specific audiences. The Australian Qualifications Framework [5] specifies that graduates with a bachelor's degree will have communication skills to present a clear, coherent and independent exposition of knowledge and ideas. Within individual programs VALUE rubrics [18] may also be adapted. These external resources can be used to promote a shared understanding of the standards for outcomes in an entire program of study.

3. Curriculum Design to Promote Outcomes around Communication in Pharmacy

The concept of the "the seven star pharmacist" developed over two decades ago proposed essential, minimum, common expectations of specific knowledge, attitudes, skills and behaviours for pharmacists. In the role of the pharmacist as a communicator, "He or she must be knowledgeable and confident while interacting with other health professionals and the public. Communication involves verbal, non-verbal, listening and writing skills" [6]. Communication skills are included in the more recently developed FIP Global Competency Framework as well as in outcome frameworks from a number of jurisdictions such as Australia, Canada, the United Kingdom, the United States [7] and the European Union [19,20]. A reported systematic search of pharmacy education literature identified that oral interpersonal communication skills and clinical writing skills were most often taught through simulated and standardised patient interactions and pharmacy practice experience courses with both subjective and objective assessments reported [21]

Identification of the relevant knowledge, skills, and attitudes that are pertinent to one aspect of communication for pharmacists, i.e., the therapeutic encounters between pharmacists and patients, has been facilitated through comparison to work in medical education which has defined elements which characterise effective communication in several clinical contexts [22], providing a coherent framework for assessing communication skills. For example, a single rubric which described four communication domains (structuring the encounter, establishes a trusting relationship, utilises effective verbal and nonverbal communication and retrieval and delivery of information) enabled the demonstration of longitudinally improving communication skills across five semesters of a pharmacy program [23].

4. Curriculum Design to Promote Outcomes around Accountability

In addition to being classified by profession-differentiated competencies, it has been suggested that all health professionals are defined as accountable practitioners [24] and indeed accountability is regarded as an essential competency of professionalism. However, accountability is an ambiguous term, often interchanged with responsibility. For the purposes of this paper accountability is defined as the continuous process of monitoring one's professional conduct, through independent thought, explaining and justifying actions, whereas responsibility traditionally means performing tasks in an accurate and timely way [25].

Learning opportunities for and assessment of accountability have been relatively neglected in the teaching and learning literature and indicators for the achievement of accountability are highly varied. Accountability has been linked to something as simple as hand washing in routine clinical practice [26] or maintaining competence and undertaking continuing professional development [27].

For students, measurable indicators have yet to be refined as can be seen from an analysis of a cross-section of recent literature described below, which specifically references the learning of accountability.

- Professional conduct and accountability has been described as being strengthened [28] through a role play exercise in process engineering in which students worked in engineering production teams. Here accountability was identified through questioning of students on all aspects of the production process, presumably demonstrating team participation with students accepting responsibility for their statements and assertions.
- Students have been encouraged to be accountable participants in their learning and actively engage in self-directed learning through planning forms for clinical placements which were assigned grades [29]. Team-based learning with specific guidelines to nursing students around "readiness" to participate has also been associated with accountability demonstrated through advanced preparation for classes or contributions to team activities [30]. A similar strategy of requiring advanced preparation for classes in flipped classrooms, where materials are provided to students outside of formal class time and using formal class time for students to undertake collaborative and interactive activities, has also been specifically associated with developing students' accountability [31].
- An enquiry-based training program for nursing students, collaboratively developed with a legal firm [32] which includes a simulated court case has been evaluated through student feedback, "Students felt that the module had strengthened their knowledge about accountable practice" [32] (p. 719), with further work from the same group substantiating the teaching approach [33].
- High-fidelity simulation cases which provide students with a realistic patient learning experience using computerised mannequins have been used to prompt nursing students to identify accountability skills and thus "may assist students in learning accountability", [34] (p. 430).

- Engineering accountability has also been taught through physical prototyping of design projects, i.e., fabrication of designs rather than production of paper designs, which are tested and verified against project objectives with the outcome of "added accountability" [35].
- In physical therapy, a curriculum innovation which included a combination of standardised patients, reflection and online communities of practice in a 360-Degree assessment loop has been described as resulting in changes to student awareness of professional core values, including accountability. In this case, accountability, which included acknowledgement and acceptance of the consequences of one's own actions, was self-assessed [36]. It is important to acknowledge that the examples cited in this paper are portions of a larger curriculum and no comment can be made regarding the accountability of the programs' graduates.

5. Curriculum Design to Promote Outcomes around Accountability in Pharmacy

World Health Organisation guidelines on good pharmacy practice make clear reference to pharmacists as professionals with responsibilities and accountabilities which include "seeking to ensure that people derive maximum therapeutic benefit from their treatments with medicines" [37]. In the United States of America, hospital pharmacists have emphasised personal accountability for their professional practice as a unifying strategy for over 50 years [38]. In Australia the current competency framework also addresses accountability, for example "Pharmacists are accountable for the services provided and the associated outcomes" [39]. The professional competencies for Canadian pharmacists at entry to practice specify "accept responsibility and accountability for own actions and decisions" [40]. This core competency is also incorporated into outcomes for students. The American Association of Colleges of Pharmacy's Center for the Advancement of Pharmacy Education (CAPE) Educational Outcomes specify accountability to both professional practice and to patients [41]. Reliability, responsibility and accountability are defined in terms of being punctual, fulfilling responsibilities in a timely and manner, following instructions, undertaking activities in a self-directed manner, demonstrating a desire to exceed expectations, demonstrating accountability and accepting responsibility for one's own actions [41]. Learning outcome statements from Australia and Canada both specify accountability towards patients [7]. As regards standards the Association of Faculties of Pharmacy of Canada Educational Outcomes Task Force provides, only one outcome description references accountability, and this is at a level below that required to graduate "violate fundamental ethical principles related to professional accountability" [14].

Learning opportunities for and the assessment of accountability in the pharmacy education literature have described team-based learning, promoted as holding students accountable for pre-class preparation [42,43]. Demonstration to students of accountability for professional actions through a patient advocacy–related curriculum using oral presentations and role play [44] has also been proposed, however not evidenced.

6. Refining Outcomes around Accountability

The literature which references the teaching and learning of accountability can be categorised in two different approaches. In the first of these approaches, students are "rewarded" explicitly through marks for the demonstration of accountability though preparation for learning activities [29,42,43], performance in teams [28,30] or adequate preparation for flipped classroom activities through low-stakes assessment [31], which do not relate specifically to professional practice. Teachers, rather than students, undertake the monitoring role and the actual transference of accountability to professional practice is unknown. "Training" is focused on the individual student being accountable to themselves, or to their team.

In the second approach, students participate in practical, simulated activities that "evoke or replicate substantial aspects of the real world" ([45] (p. i2), [44]). Learning of accountability is "evidenced" through students being able to identify accountability through these activities [32–34] or anticipated by academic staff [35]. No explicit reference is made to measure of achieving accountability [32–35] and, again, actual transference of accountability to professional practice post-graduation is unknown. In this case, students are exposed to concepts of accountability to their patients or clients and the community.

Thus, although the curriculum has been described as being focused on accountability, it is in fact focused on accountability to the self, to the team or accountability to patients/clients. The curriculum examples cited in this paper are displayed according to the focus of the sphere of influence for curriculum innovation, i.e., self, team, patient/client and the broader health system, in Figure 1.

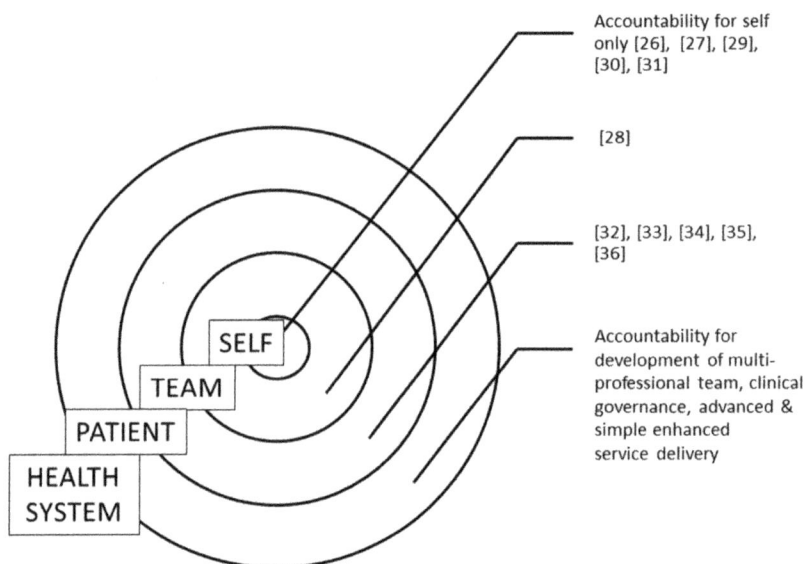

Figure 1. Examples of teaching and assessment of accountability from literature mapped according to sphere of influence.

7. Discussion

Identification of appropriate indicators for the achievement of a desired competence is critical to being able to assess student outcomes. In the case of communication clear outcomes, teaching approaches and assessment are regularly described in the literature. Consideration by university teachers of the appropriate sphere of influence for a student will facilitate clarification of the outcome as accountability to the self, to the team, to patients/clients or indeed to the broader health system and the development of both teaching and assessment activities appropriate for each student cohort. This consideration means that the outcome accountability may be refined, for example, "students are accountable for pre-class preparation", and learning activities and assessment consequently focused explicitly on accountability to the self.

8. Conclusions

Identifying appropriate teaching approaches and assessments depends upon the desired outcomes. This paper presents a comparison between the outcomes of accountability and communication. In the case of communication, outcomes are clearly defined and resources are available to inform teaching and assessment of communication. However, in the case of the critical outcome accountability, valid and reliable assessments and approaches to the teaching of accountability are yet to be developed. Figure 1 displays examples of accountability teaching and learning from the literature mapped according to the sphere of influence of an individual student. This paper adds to the literature by providing a model which may be useful for teaching staff considering teaching and assessment activities around the critical competence of accountability.

This paper has focused on outcomes as being central to students' achievement. However, it is important to acknowledge that there are other factors which affect student learning and determine whether students develop the requisite outcomes, for example the approaches educators use to design and teach courses.

Conflicts of Interest: The author declares no conflict of interest.

References

1. Lenburg, C.B. The framework, concepts and methods of the competency outcomes and performance assessment (COPA) model. *Online J. Issues Nurs.* **1999**, *4*, 1–12.
2. Biggs, J.; Tang, C. *Teaching for Quality learning at University: What the Student Does*, 3rd ed.; Open University Press: Maidenhead, UK, 2007.
3. European Association for Quality Assurance in Higher Education. *Standards and Guidelines for Quality Assurance in the European Higher Education Area*; European Higher Education Area: Helsinki, Finland, 2005.
4. Lumina Foundation. *The Degree Qualifications Profile*; Lumina Foundation: Indianapolis, IN, USA, 2011.
5. Australian Qualifications Framework, (N.D.). AQF Qualification by Sector of Accreditation. Available online: http://www.aqf.edu.au/Portals/0/Documents/Handbook/AQF_Handbook_51-72.pdf (accessed on 24 June 2016).
6. World Health Organisation. The Role of the Pharmacist in the Health Care System. 1997. Available online: http://apps.who.int/medicinedocs/en/d/Js2214e/3.2.html#Js2214e.3.2 (accessed on 24 June 2016).
7. Stupans, I.; Atkinson, J.; Meštrović, A.; Nash, R.; Rouse, M.J. A Shared Focus: Comparing the Australian, Canadian, United Kingdom and United States Pharmacy Learning Outcome Frameworks and the Global Competency Framework. *Pharmacy* **2016**, *4*, 26. [CrossRef]
8. Kennedy, D. *Writing and Using Learning Outcomes: A Practical Guide*; University College Cork: Cork, Ireland, 2006.
9. Spitzberg, B.H. Communication Competence as Knowledge, Skill, and Impression. *Commun. Educ.* **1983**, *32*, 323–329. [CrossRef]
10. Anderson, L.W.; Krathwohl, C.R.; Airasian, P.W.; Cruikshank, K.A. (Eds.) *A Taxonomy for Learning, Teaching, and Assessing—A Revision of Bloom's Taxonomy of Educational Objectives*; Addison Wesley Longman: New York, NY, USA, 2001.
11. Mead, N.A.; Rubin, D.L. *Assessing Listening and Speaking Skills*; ERIC Clearinghouse: Washington, DC, USA, 1985.
12. Benner, P. Using the Dreyfus model of skill acquisition to describe and interpret skill acquisition and clinical judgment in nursing practice and education. *Bull. Sci. Technol. Soc.* **2004**, *24*, 188–199. [CrossRef]
13. Dreyfus, S.E. The five-stage model of adult skill acquisition. *Bull. Sci. Technol. Soc.* **2004**, *24*, 177–181. [CrossRef]
14. Brown, T.; Brown, T.; Mailhot, C.; Schindel, T.; Waite, N. *Levels of Performance Expected of Students Graduating from First Professional Degree Programs in Pharmacy in Canada*; Association of Faculties of Pharmacy of Canada: Ottawa, ON, Canada, 2011.
15. Reddy, Y.M.; Andrade, H. A review of rubric use in higher education. *Assess. Eval. High. Educ.* **2010**, *35*, 435–448. [CrossRef]
16. Dawson, P. Assessment rubrics: Towards clearer and more replicable design, research and practice. *Assess. Eval. High. Educ.* **2017**, *42*, 347–360. [CrossRef]
17. Jonsson, A.; Svingby, G. The use of scoring rubrics: Reliability, validity and educational consequences. *Educ. Res. Rev.* **2007**, *2*, 130–144. [CrossRef]
18. Association of American Colleges and Universities Rubrics. 2010. Available online: http://www.aacu.org/value/index.cfm (accessed on 24 June 2016).
19. Atkinson, J.; de Paepe, K.; Pozo, A.S.; Rekkas, D.; Volmer, D.; Hirvonen, J.; Bozic, B.; Skowron, A.; Mircioiu, C.; Marcincal, A.; et al. The PHAR-QA Project: Competency framework for pharmacy practice—First steps, the results of the European network Delphi Round 1. *Pharmacy* **2015**, *3*, 307–329. [CrossRef]

20. Atkinson, J.; de Paepe, K.; Pozo, A.S.; Rekkas, D.; Volmer, D.; Hirvonen, J.; Bozic, B.; Skowron, A.; Mircioiu, C.; Marcincal, A.; et al. The Second Round of the PHAR-QA Survey of Competences for Pharmacy Practice. *Pharmacy* **2016**, *4*, 27. [CrossRef]

21. Wallman, A.; Vaudan, C.; Sporrong, S.K. Communications training in pharmacy education, 1995–2010. *Am. J. Pharm. Educ.* **2013**, *77*, 36. [CrossRef] [PubMed]

22. Makoul, G. Essential elements of communication in medical encounters: The Kalamazoo consensus statement. *Acad. Med.* **2001**, *76*, 390–393. [CrossRef] [PubMed]

23. Thompson, M.; Gilliam, E.; Nuffer, W. Longitudinal assessment of students' communication and professionalism skills across all levels of a Pharm D curriculum. *J. Pharm. Care Health Syst.* **2015**. [CrossRef]

24. Frenk, J.; Chen, L.; Bhutta, Z.A.; Cohen, J.; Crisp, N.; Evans, T.; Fineberg, H.; Garcia, P.; Ke, Y.; Kelley, P.; et al. Health professionals for a new century: transforming education to strengthen health systems in an interdependent world. *Lancet* **2010**, *376*, 1923–1958. [CrossRef]

25. Savage, J. *Interpreting Accountability: An Ethnographic Study of Practice Nurses, Accountability and Multidisciplinary Team Decision-Making in the Context of Clinical Governance*; Royal College of Nursing: London, UK, 2004.

26. Goldmann, D. System failure versus personal accountability—The case for clean hands. *N. Engl. J. Med.* **2006**, *355*, 121–123. [CrossRef] [PubMed]

27. Scrivener, R.; Hooper, R. Accountability and responsibility: Principle of nursing practice B. *Nurs. Stand.* **2011**, *25*, 35–36. [CrossRef] [PubMed]

28. Raineya, T.; Jayasuriyab, K.; Gottlieba, U. Integrating 'role play' in assessment to strengthen professional conduct and accountability of students: A pilot study. In Proceedings of the Annual Conference of the Australasian Association for Engineering Education, Wellington, New Zealand, 8–10 December 2014.

29. Brown, D.L.; Ferrill, M.J.; Hinton, A.B.; Shek, A. Self-Directed Professional Development: The Pursuit of Affective Learning. *Am. J. Pharm. Educ.* **2001**, *65*, 240–246.

30. Mennenga, H.A. Team-Based Learning: Engagement and Accountability with Psychometric Analysis of a New Instrument. Ph.D. Thesis, University of Nevada, Las Vegas, NV, USA, 2010.

31. Gilboy, M.B.; Heinerichs, S.; Pazzaglia, G. Enhancing Student Engagement Using the Flipped Classroom. *J. Nutr. Educ. Behav.* **2015**, *47*, 109–114. [CrossRef] [PubMed]

32. Plant, N.; Pitt, R.; Troke, B. A partnership approach to learning about accountability. *Br. J. Nurs.* **2010**, *19*, 718–719. [CrossRef] [PubMed]

33. Pitt, R.; Narayanasamy, A.; Plant, N. An evaluation of teaching and learning accountable practice in nurse education. *J. Furth. High. Educ.* **2015**, *40*, 612–629. [CrossRef]

34. Bussard, M.E. High-Fidelity Simulation to Teach Accountability to Prelicensure Nursing Students. *Clin. Simul. Nurs.* **2015**, *11*, 425–430. [CrossRef]

35. Retzlaff, R.; Torvi, D.; Burton, R. Teaching Engineering Accountability through Physical Prototyping. In Proceedings of the Canadian Engineering Education Association, Canmore, AB, Canada, 8–11 June 2014.

36. Hayward, L.M.; Blackmer, B. A model for teaching and assessing core values development in doctor of physical therapy students. *J. Phys. Ther. Educ.* **2010**, *24*, 16.

37. World Health Organization. *Joint FIP/WHO Guidelines on Good Pharmacy Practice: Standards for Quality of Pharmacy Services*; WHO Technical Report Series; World Health Organization: Geneva, Switzerland, 2011.

38. Weber, R.; Stevenson, J.; Ng, C.; White, S. Measuring change in health-system pharmacy over 50 years: "Reflecting" on the Mirror, Part I. *Hosp. Pharm.* **2013**, *48*, 966–969. [CrossRef] [PubMed]

39. Pharmaceutical Society of Australia. *Competency Standards for Pharmacists in Australia*; Pharmaceutical Society of Australia: Canberra, Australia, 2010.

40. National Association of Pharmacy Regulatory Authorities. *Professional Competencies for Canadian Pharmacists at Entry to Practice*; National Association of Pharmacy Regulatory Authorities: Ottawa, ON, Canada, 2014.

41. Medina, M.S.; Plaza, C.M.; Stowe, C.D.; Robinson, E.T.; DeLander, G.; Beck, D.E.; Melchert, R.B.; Supernaw, R.B.; Roche, V.F.; Gleason, B.L.; et al. Center for the Advancement of Pharmacy Education 2013 educational outcomes. *Am. J. Pharm. Educ.* **2013**, *77*, 162. [CrossRef] [PubMed]

42. Ofstad, W.; Brunner, L.J. Team-based learning in pharmacy education. *Am. J. Pharm. Educ.* **2013**, *77*, 70. [CrossRef] [PubMed]

43. Tejada, F.R.; Fasanella, D.R.; Elfadaly, M. Students' Opinions on Summative Team Assessments in a Three-Year Concentrated Pharmacy Curriculum. *Am. J. Pharm. Educ.* **2016**, *80*, 103. [PubMed]

44. Mraiche, F.; Paravattil, B.; Wilby, K.J. The use of oral presentations, role-play sessions, and reflective critiques to emphasize the advocate learning outcome in the pharmacy curriculum. *Curr. Pharm. Teach. Learn.* **2015**, *7*, 443–450. [CrossRef]

45. Gaba, D.M. The future vision of simulation in health care. *Qual. Saf. Health Care* **2004**, *13* (Suppl. 1), i2–i10. [CrossRef] [PubMed]

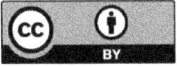

pharmacy

MDPI

Review

Implementation of Competency-Based Pharmacy Education (CBPE)

Andries Koster [1],*, Tom Schalekamp [2] and Irma Meijerman [3]

[1] Department of Pharmaceutical Sciences, Utrecht University, The Netherlands and European Association of Faculties of Pharmacy (EAFP), Utrecht 3508 TB, The Netherlands
[2] Department of Pharmaceutical Sciences, Utrecht University, Utrecht 3508 TB, The Netherlands; T.Schalekamp@uu.nl
[3] Department of Pharmaceutical Sciences, The Netherlands and Centre for Teaching and Learning, Utrecht University, Utrecht 3508 TB, The Netherlands; I.Meijerman@uu.nl
* Correspondence: A.S.Koster@uu.nl; Tel.: +31-30-2537353

Academic Editor: Jeffrey Atkinson
Received: 4 January 2017; Accepted: 16 February 2017; Published: 21 February 2017

Abstract: Implementation of competency-based pharmacy education (CBPE) is a time-consuming, complicated process, which requires agreement on the tasks of a pharmacist, commitment, institutional stability, and a goal-directed developmental perspective of all stakeholders involved. In this article the main steps in the development of a fully-developed competency-based pharmacy curriculum (bachelor, master) are described and tips are given for a successful implementation. After the choice for entering into CBPE is made and a competency framework is adopted (step 1), intended learning outcomes are defined (step 2), followed by analyzing the required developmental trajectory (step 3) and the selection of appropriate assessment methods (step 4). Designing the teaching-learning environment involves the selection of learning activities, student experiences, and instructional methods (step 5). Finally, an iterative process of evaluation and adjustment of individual courses, and the curriculum as a whole, is entered (step 6). Successful implementation of CBPE requires a system of effective quality management and continuous professional development as a teacher. In this article suggestions for the organization of CBPE and references to more detailed literature are given, hoping to facilitate the implementation of CBPE.

Keywords: assessment; competence; competency-based education; constructive alignment; curriculum; development; entrustable professional activity; learning outcomes

---

1. Introduction

> *If you want to grow a worthwhile plant: a rose, a fruit tree, a vine of paan, then you need effort.*
>
> > *You must water, apply manure, weed it, prune it.*
>
> *It is not simple.*
>
> > *So it is with the world.*

Vikram Seth: A suitable boy

National and international tendencies indicate that competency-based educational models are becoming dominant for the education of heath care professionals, such as nursing [1], dentistry [2], medicine [3], and pharmacy [4,5]. The main driver for adopting competency-based educational designs is the need to prepare pharmacists for their societal role, ultimately leading to improvement of health care and patient safety [6–9]. However, implementation of a competency-base pharmacy curriculum is a formidable task, in particular if an existing curriculum is organized in a disciplinary, content-driven, teacher-centered way, in which students are expected to mainly attend lectures and to perform in well-structured practical exercises reproducing compounding and analytical tasks as described in national formularies of pharmacopoeias. Even though this description of a 'traditional' curriculum can be considered stereotypical, most readers will recognize elements of this description in their local pharmacy curricula. An additional problem in developing a pharmacy curriculum is the recent change in the tasks of the pharmacist, which, during the last decades, has shown a shift from product-orientation to more patient-orientation (FIP 2012, [4]). Transforming a 'traditional' educational practice into competency-based pharmacy education (CBPE), which pays attention to both the science-based and patient-oriented aspects of pharmacy in a balanced way, will involve re-thinking of the roles of teachers, the roles of students, and re-designing of assessment tasks and many educational activities [10,11]. Moreover, a pharmacy department or faculty is usually organized along disciplines ranging from medicinal chemistry, via biopharmacy to pharmacotherapeutics and social pharmacy. It is, therefore, necessary to create a curriculum management structure and a human resources allocation model, which may interfere or conflict with existing hierarchies and research interests.

This paper describes the essential steps in designing a competency-based pharmacy curriculum and gives tips for a successful organization, development, and implementation of such curricula. Suggestions will be based on literature references whenever possible, but will also be 'colored' by the authors' experiences with implementing new curricula in the field of pharmacy and pharmaceutical sciences [12,13]. Readers should be aware that the possibility to make radical changes in existing curricula depend heavily on the local situation, in particular with respect to the experienced need for change, the preparedness to embark on a complicated journey, and the willingness of the formal departmental and/or university structure to support and facilitate the change process. The experiences of the authors are 'colored' by the way a curriculum renewal was handled in a positive and stimulating way by the departmental leadership (cf. [14]). It is, therefore, uncertain whether all aspects, which refer to the authors' own experiences, can be easily implemented in other environments. Nevertheless, we hope that this article can be a guide in starting an interesting journey towards competency-based pharmacy education (CBPE).

2. Competency-Based Pharmacy Education

The attention for competency-based pharmacy education is relatively recent, compared to other health care professional programs. The American Association of Colleges of Pharmacy has pioneered the development of educational outcome-based guidelines since the early 1990s (AACP 2013, [10]) and a global competency framework was published by the International Pharmaceutical Federation more recently (FIP 2012, [4]). Descriptions of the entry-into-practice requirements for professional pharmacists are available for Canada (AFPC 2010), the United Kingdom (GPhC 2011), Australia (NCSF 2010 [15]), and Europe (EPCF 2016, [9]). These descriptions can be based on different models and may have more or less official legal status, but they all intend to function as guiding principles for the evaluation and 're-engineering' of existing curricula and the design and development of new curricula. The requirements for entry-level pharmacists are usually defined in terms of learning outcomes or competencies and are ordered on the basis of Miller's pyramid of clinical competence [16]. The diversity of frameworks (see Appendix A) illustrates that no 'golden standard' for a competency framework exists. As long as the framework is internally consistent and captures all aspects of the required professional competence, it can be used as a tool for the analysis, development, and structuring of a curriculum. Existing frameworks for pharmacy education appear to be similar across jurisdictions [17] and health care competency frameworks in general appear to address the same aspects of professional competence. The use of competency standards for undergraduate pharmacy education was recently reviewed by Nash et al. [5].

Apart from competency frameworks covering the complete initial Pharmacy higher education program, competency profiles have been developed for separate curriculum domains, e.g., advanced pharmacy practice [18], professional development skills [19], or related specialization areas, such as clinical pharmacology [20] or pharmaceutical medicine [21].

3. Terminology and Definitions

The implementation of CBPE is often complicated by concepts and terminology, which is experienced as ill-defined or confusing [22,23]. Medical competence is defined as "The array of abilities across multiple domains or aspects of physician performance in a certain context. Statements about competence require descriptive qualifiers to define the relevant abilities, context, and stage of training. Competence is multi-dimensional and dynamic. It changes with time, experience, and setting" (cited from [3], (p. 641)). We suggest that the same definition can be used for other health care professionals, including pharmacists, by changing the use of 'physician' into any other relevant professional job description.

The definition of competence makes clear that competence of a student or pharmacist can only be observed or assessed in the context of specific well-defined circumstances. Being competent in one professional situation does not necessarily imply competence in another situation (competence is *contextual*), and students need time to become competent in different aspects of their intended profession (competence is *developmental*). Moreover, it is highly unlikely that all students can acquire competence at the same rate and with the same amount of training provided; large inter-individual differences are usually encountered. Finally, competence is only demonstrated when all relevant knowledge, skills, and behavior is used in an integrated way which is relevant in a particular professional situation (competence is *multidimensional*). The contextual, developmental, and multidimensional nature of the competence to be achieved by a curriculum has important consequences for the organization of CBPE, in particular with respect to assessment and progression of students through the curriculum [3,24].

An approach to deal with the complex nature of CBPE is to use *entrustable professional activities* (EPAs) for the operationalization of educational outcomes at the transition of undergraduate education to professional working life. EPAs are carefully described aspects of professional acting, respecting the contextual and developmental aspects of competence, which are used to structure learning, training, and assessment of starting professionals enrolled in medical specialization programs [23]. By proposing the use of EPAs as a way of structuring medical education at an earlier stage, the undergraduate curriculum, medical educators intend to ease the abrupt transition from undergraduate to graduate education [24]. In this conception, undergraduate education, entry into professional life, further specialization, and postgraduate training become a flexible educational continuum where training and assessment is structured by using EPAs as building blocks of competence. In the context of pharmacy education, EPAs are used for structuring the advanced pharmacy practice experience of the University of Minnesota College of Pharmacy, USA [25] and the postgraduate 'advanced community pharmacy' specialization in the Netherlands [26].

Competence can be conceptualized as consisting of various ingredients, or building blocks, which together enables the student to function in a competent way. These building blocks of competence are designated as competencies (singular: *competency*). Competencies are preferably specified as observable abilities of a pharmacist, integrating multiple components such as knowledge, skills, values, and attitudes, and expressed as actual behavior. Since competencies are observable, they can be measured and assessed to ensure that students have acquired them [3]. Moreover, progression of students through the curriculum can be guided and monitored by defining intermediate stages in the acquirement of competencies (see below). These intermediate stages can be used as anchor points to structure the curriculum and/or as critical points for assessing whether students are progressing according to expectations. Competencies are acquired by the students while they progress through the curriculum and must be considered a personal qualities or abilities of the student [23].

In order to guide the development of assessment formats and teaching-learning activities (see below) competencies usually need to be further broken down in their constituent elements.

Most competencies, as defined in existing competency frameworks, each consist of a unique mixture of knowledge in particular disciplines, cognitive skills, non-cognitive skills, and attitudinal aspects, which need to be used or applied in an integrated way. In undergraduate education different fields of knowledge (disciplinary or otherwise) and a variety of skills (technical, cognitive, non-cognitive, etc.) can be taught or trained in several ways, but assessment is largely done with dedicated assessment formats, which are aimed at capturing specific learning objectives. The results of assessments can be considered the observable *learning outcome* of competency-based education and are defined in terms of knowledge, skills, and behavior. Intended learning outcomes are preferably described with action verbs, which indicate the required cognitive level. Furthermore, the conditions under which the concrete behavior is expected to be demonstrated, must be specified in the intended learning outcomes [27,28]. Examples of intended learning outcomes for a content domain and for a generic skill are given below (Section 5). Learning outcomes can be ordered in different domains and different developmental stages to guide curriculum development.

In the previous paragraph the term 'learning outcome' is used in a specific sense to describe the results of assessment of the knowledge and skills elements of individual competencies; a learning outcome in this case is subordinate to a competency. It must be remarked that in the literature the term 'learning outcome' is also used in a more general way to describe the results of an educational program at different levels of integration; acquired competencies and entrusted professional activities can also be described as learning outcomes [15,22].

4. Curriculum Design Process

The design of a competency-based curriculum ideally follows a specific sequence from competencies to learning outcomes, to assessments, to teaching-learning activities. This process can be described in six steps (Figure 1, adapted from [3]). Depending on the local situation, a curriculum change process can be more or less challenging, and success or failure will depend on the felt sense of urgency, the creation of a shared explicit vision on the future, and the willingness of all participants to engage in discussing fundamental issues, related to scientific identity and societal responsibility. Involvement of a diversity of stakeholders, both within and outside academia, and a careful 'orchestration' of the change process is necessary [29,30]. In our experience a combination of strong external pressure (e.g., a critical visitation or a critical attitude of professional organizations), internal dissatisfaction with the existing educational quality (often latent among teachers, students, and alumni), and courage of the institutional leadership to make a fundamental change, will make transformation from a 'traditional' curriculum to a competency-based curriculum possible. Even then, it is advised to monitor the change process carefully and to be aware of the socio-political aspects of the way the change process is organized [29].

Once a decision is made to embark on the journey to CBPE, the first two steps (Figure 1) are mainly strategic and intend to position the curriculum in the local context. The first step can be complex because the pharmacy profession has evolved from a nearly exclusively product-orientation to a more patient-orientation. Within a faculty or department a certain degree of consensus must be reached on the consequences of this shift, which necessitates more attention to softer disciplines such as pharmacotherapeutics and patient counselling, including communication skills. A pitfall in the first curriculum development step can be the introduction of new disciplines and new skills without reducing more traditional ones, resulting in overburdening the curriculum. Moreover, the main driving force for a curriculum rebuilding must be the learning process of the students and the responsibility to educate them to competent professionals, who can function adequately in the context of the local health care system or the local pharmaceutical research environment [16,31]. This means that—even though competency frameworks can be used as guidelines—interpretation and fine-tuning of the required competencies and competence levels is necessary. Another aspect is the need to consider accommodating a certain degree of specialization or profiling within the curriculum. The result of the strategic choices made will be a description of competencies and learning outcomes, which is more detailed than the general framework used as a starting point. Several examples of curriculum implementations in different contexts can be found in the literature (see Table 1).

- **Tip 1: Use a competency framework.** Several competency frameworks are available (see Appendix A). All can be used as a starting point for curriculum development but interpretation and fine-tuning to the local situation is necessary.
- **Tip 2: Consult all your stakeholders.** In designing a new curriculum consultation of the outside world is necessary to align the competences of recent graduates to the local professional and healthcare needs.
- **Tip 3: Think forward (scenarios).** Curriculum changes are usually implemented gradually, starting from the first year of the program. This means, that your newly-educated graduates will enter practice at least five years from now!

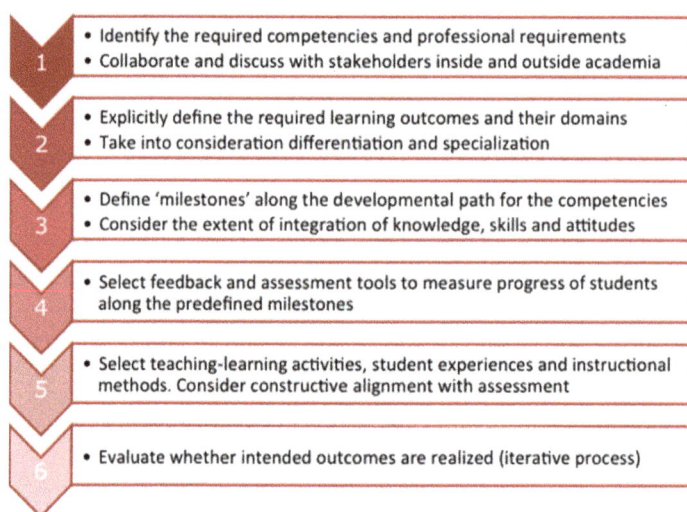

1
- Identify the required competencies and professional requirements
- Collaborate and discuss with stakeholders inside and outside academia

2
- Explicitly define the required learning outcomes and their domains
- Take into consideration differentiation and specialization

3
- Define 'milestones' along the developmental path for the competencies
- Consider the extent of integration of knowledge, skills and attitudes

4
- Select feedback and assessment tools to measure progress of students along the predefined milestones

5
- Select teaching-learning activities, student experiences and instructional methods. Consider constructive alignment with assessment

6
- Evaluate whether intended outcomes are realized (iterative process)

Figure 1. The curriculum design process.

Table 1. Examples of curriculum design and construction.

Curriculum	Description	Reference
B.Sc.	Content and generic skills for a pre-professional curriculum (nationwide, USA)	[32]
B.Pharm.	Design of an outcomes-based Pharmacy curriculum (Hong-Kong, China)	[33]
B.Pharm.Sc.	Undergraduate honours programme for the training of pharmaceutical researchers (Utrecht, the Netherlands)	[12]
Pharm.D.	An integrated professional pharmacy curriculum (Denver, USA)	[34]
B.Sc. + M.Sc.	Design of a complete bachelor and master programme (Helsinki, Finland)	[31]
Ph.D.	Research training for clinical pharmaceutical sciences: assessments and rubrics (Pittsburgh, USA)	[35]
M.D.	Content and skills for the core curriculum of a medical school (Sheffield, United Kingdom)	[36]
M.D.	Teaching, training, and assessment of professional behaviour in medicine (Amsterdam, The Netherlands)	[37]
Physician assistants	Teaching, training and assessment for physician assistants (Utrecht, The Netherlands)	[38]

5. Curriculum Construction

Step 3 of the curriculum implementation process (Figure 1) is a crucial one. A competency-based curriculum is much more than a collection of courses: curricular elements, such as individual courses, (research) projects and pharmacy practice placements need to be organized in a logical sequence and decisions must be made about the obligatory or elective nature of the elements, taking into account possible specializations or profiling of students during the curriculum. It is helpful to explicitly formulate principles for the curriculum construction, which can serve as an internal 'frame of reference' or 'reflection tool' for steering and adjusting the construction process. Sharing these principles with teachers, students, and others involved in the curriculum implementation can ease the development process. In Table 2 an example is given of the principles that we have used during the curriculum design process at Utrecht University in the past.

Table 2. Seven principles for design and construction of a curriculum.

1	The curriculum is designed as a coherent program.
2	The program stimulates active study behaviour, is challenging and varied.
3	Acquisition, application and integration of knowledge and skills take place in a context relevant for the future profession.
4	Within the program systematic and explicit attention is paid to the development of academic and personal skills and values.
5	Direction of the learning process is gradually shifted from teacher to student.
6	The program enables students to follow individual interests by offering elective courses and a patient- or product-oriented profile.
7	A well-balanced system of mentoring and assessment is used, which takes into account the steering effects of testing.

Example of guiding principles used for the design of a new pharmacy curriculum (bachelor, master) at Utrecht University in 2001, cited from [13].

Two aspects of the curriculum design need further attention: integration of content and skills in curricular elements and the longitudinal development of knowledge and skills, also described as horizontal and vertical integration, respectively [11]. The first aspect—integration of knowledge and skills—is a fundamental requirement in CBPE because students are expected to acquire complex competences during their study, where the required knowledge, cognitive and non-cognitive skills are expected to be used in an integrated way (AACP 2013, AFPC 2010, [11]). For the design of a competency-based curriculum this raises the question where, when, and how integration can be realized. In traditional curricula the change from non-integrated to integrated learning can be very abrupt, usually when a student is confronted with pharmacy practice for the first time, either during rotations or entry into professional practice. In less traditional curricula a more gradual approach, where students are moving from learning skills in isolation to application of skills in the context of professionally relevant tasks—with a gradual increase in complexity—is advocated [11,39]. This can be achieved by using problem-based and project-based learning methods of a relatively restricted nature in early phases of the curriculum, and a gradual increase in the complexity of assignments or projects as the curriculum progresses [12]. In later stages of the curriculum, simulations of pharmacy practice (e.g., the pharmacy game Gimmics®, [40]) and organizing the curriculum around EPAs (see above) can train students in real-life pharmacy practice situations under complex, but still safe and supervised, conditions without giving students full responsibility.

A gradual increase in the extent of integration of skills as the curriculum progresses requires that the development of skills and their integration with the content of the curriculum is explicitly analyzed and translated into teaching and learning activities, which confront students with challenging tasks during the whole curriculum. This requires that knowledge about the learning of skills must be present among the teachers and that some overarching description is available of the way development of skills is organized, monitored and assessed. In our situation in Utrecht this is realized by making selected teachers responsible for the development of different skills tracks, such as 'pharmaceutical calculations', 'compounding', 'research methodology', 'oral communication', and 'written communication'. These teachers are stimulated to specialize in these didactic areas and participate in local networks with teachers from other faculties or universities. Within the pharmacy program, they function as consultants to the teachers who are responsible for the different courses of the curriculum. Similar track or stream coordination functions have been described for other curricula [31,41,42].

Analogous to the progression of skills, the development of content knowledge in the curriculum requires an explicit analysis of the way knowledge in different curricular domains is built up during the curriculum. These analyses can be used to explicitly formulate learning outcomes, which students are expected to have reached at intermediate stages of the curriculum. Once these intermediate stages (or 'milestones') are described, they can be used to inspire student assessment formats and guide the definition of actual course content on different levels of the curriculum. Examples of explicit intended learning outcomes at intermediate stages (end of year one, bachelor degree, and master degree) for a content domain and a skills domain of a curriculum are given in Figures 2 and 3. In the example of the content domain 'pharmacokinetics' (Figure 2), the gradual built up of knowledge from basic concepts to practice-oriented applications is illustrated. In the example of the skills domain 'oral communication' (Figure 3), it can be seen that the requirements gradually increase in complexity and that some profiling is specified during the master phase.

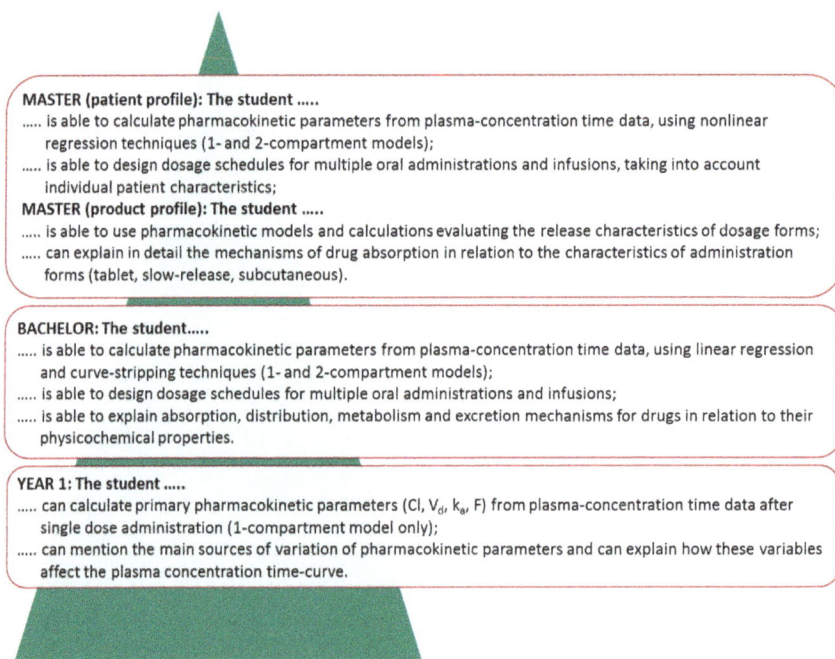

MASTER (patient profile): The student .....
..... is able to calculate pharmacokinetic parameters from plasma-concentration time data, using nonlinear regression techniques (1- and 2-compartment models);
..... is able to design dosage schedules for multiple oral administrations and infusions, taking into account individual patient characteristics;
MASTER (product profile): The student .....
..... is able to use pharmacokinetic models and calculations evaluating the release characteristics of dosage forms;
..... can explain in detail the mechanisms of drug absorption in relation to the characteristics of administration forms (tablet, slow-release, subcutaneous).

BACHELOR: The student.....
..... is able to calculate pharmacokinetic parameters from plasma-concentration time data, using linear regression and curve-stripping techniques (1- and 2-compartment models);
..... is able to design dosage schedules for multiple oral administrations and infusions;
..... is able to explain absorption, distribution, metabolism and excretion mechanisms for drugs in relation to their physicochemical properties.

YEAR 1: The student .....
..... can calculate primary pharmacokinetic parameters (Cl, V_d, k_a, F) from plasma-concentration time data after single dose administration (1-compartment model only);
..... can mention the main sources of variation of pharmacokinetic parameters and can explain how these variables affect the plasma concentration time-curve.

Figure 2. Example of curriculum layers for a content domain. Learning outcomes for the domain 'pharmacokinetics' at intermediate stages of the pharmacy curriculum in Utrecht. In this curriculum nine different content domains are distinguished, and learning outcomes are specified for the end of year one, for the bachelor degree, and for the master degree.

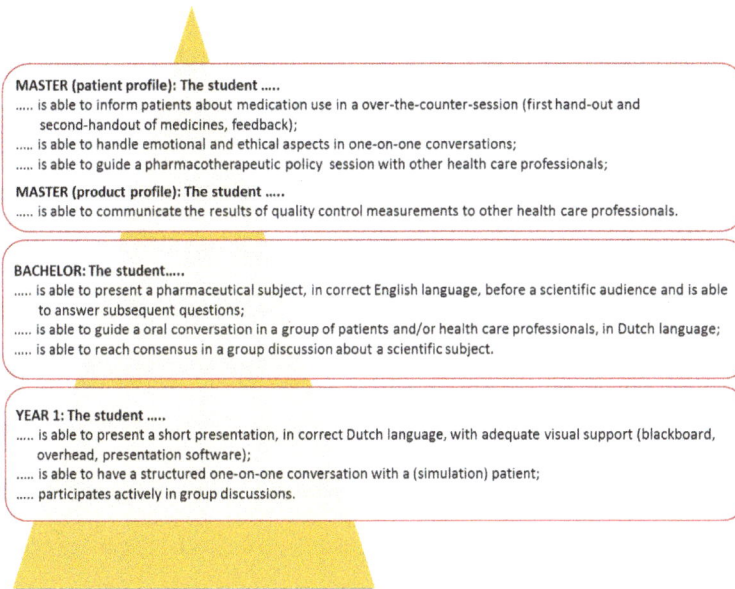

MASTER (patient profile): The student .....
..... is able to inform patients about medication use in a over-the-counter-session (first hand-out and second-handout of medicines, feedback);
..... is able to handle emotional and ethical aspects in one-on-one conversations;
..... is able to guide a pharmacotherapeutic policy session with other health care professionals;

MASTER (product profile): The student .....
..... is able to communicate the results of quality control measurements to other health care professionals.

BACHELOR: The student.....
..... is able to present a pharmaceutical subject, in correct English language, before a scientific audience and is able to answer subsequent questions;
..... is able to guide a oral conversation in a group of patients and/or health care professionals, in Dutch language;
..... is able to reach consensus in a group discussion about a scientific subject.

YEAR 1: The student .....
..... is able to present a short presentation, in correct Dutch language, with adequate visual support (blackboard, overhead, presentation software);
..... is able to have a structured one-on-one conversation with a (simulation) patient;
..... participates actively in group discussions.

Figure 3. Example of curriculum layers for a skills domain. Learning outcomes for the skill 'oral communication' at intermediate stages of the pharmacy curriculum in Utrecht. In this curriculum nine different skills domains are distinguished in total, and learning outcomes are specified for the end of year one, for the bachelor degree, and for the master degree.

Designing a curriculum is essentially a creative process, which requires the contribution of variously-minded individuals, and is best done with a combination of teachers, students, educational specialists, and administrative support personnel. Both creative, bird-like, leaders and meticulous, ant-like, workers are needed in different stages of the process [29]. In our experience, this can be organized as a curriculum committee with a flexible structure where sub-tasks can be allocated to smaller subsets of the committee as the need arises (see also [29]). Descriptions of available curriculum design processes may function as an inspiration for the reader [12,33,34,36].

- **Tip 4: Integrate content and skills as far as possible.** Skills can initially be trained in isolation, but must be integrated with course content as the curriculum advances. Professional activities usually require that knowledge, cognitive skills, and non-cognitive skills are used in an integrated way.
- **Tip 5: Appoint curriculum coordinators.** CBPE requires that the longitudinal development of knowledge and skills progresses gradually from relatively simple and isolated to more complex and integrated. This requires monitoring and readjustment of the curriculum structure by skills consultants and/or stream coordinators.

6. Student Assessment

In the next step of the implementation process (step 4 in Figure 1) formats for the summative and formative assessment of students are designed [43,44]. The goal of summative assessment (or: assessment *of* learning) is to evaluate and grade students at the end of the different curricular elements by comparing it to some standard or benchmark. The overall purpose of summative assessments in a curriculum is to guarantee that each individual student has fulfilled the curricular requirements. In the context of CBPE this means that the total of summative assessments is supposed to be representative for all required competencies. As a consequence, the student can be considered 'competent' at the level specified by the description of the required degree competencies.

The goal of formative assessment is different. Formative assessment (or: assessment *for* learning) is intended to monitor student learning, and to inform teachers and students about progress in the learning process. Formative assessment essentially has a feedback purpose and can help students to identify their strengths and weaknesses and to identify areas that need additional attention. The results of formative assessments can help teachers to identify areas which appear to be problematic for students, and can help them to adapt and improve their teaching.

Designing assessment tasks, which have a clear relation to the required competencies in CBPE, is a challenging task [22,45]. As the focus in CBPE, compared to more traditional educational formats, is strongly emphasizing the development of student abilities [3], authentic assessment tasks are called for. Authentic assessment tasks mimic aspects of the future professional life of the students and can greatly contribute to student motivation. As the curriculum progresses, assessment tasks can increase in complexity to maintain consistency with the gradual evolution of the curriculum in the direction of professional identity (illustrated in Figure 4; see also [16,24,25]). In order to maintain student motivation and to prevent student burnout, overburdening the curriculum with multiple summative assessments should be prevented. In our experience it is better to concentrate on a limited number of well-chosen summative assessments, and invest more in frequent formative assessments. Spreading assessment periods over the study year and making assessment an integral part of curricular elements (courses, projects, rotations) results in a system of 'continuous assessment', which improves study behavior and minimizes test anxiety and student burnout. Investing in the development of formative assessment tasks emphasizes the function of assessment-for-learning (formative), rather than the function of assessment-of-learning (summative) [44,45].

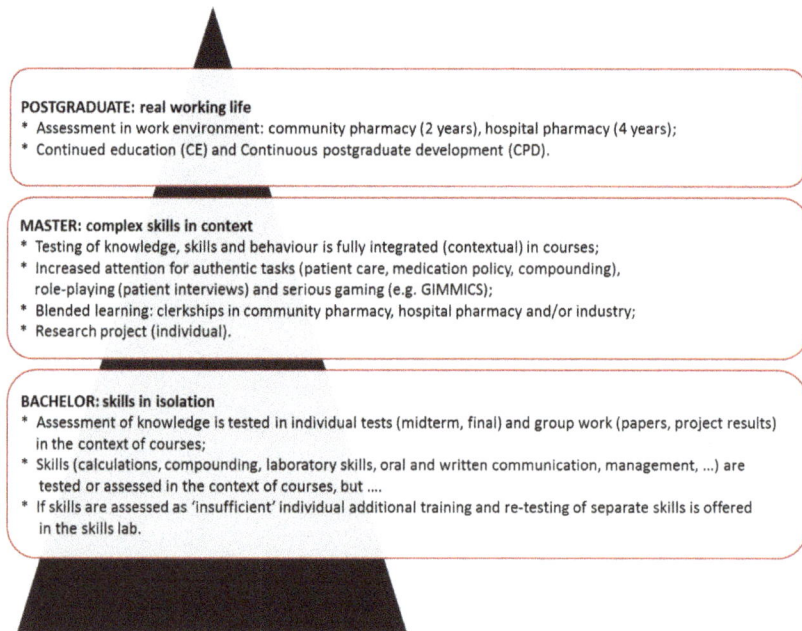

POSTGRADUATE: real working life
* Assessment in work environment: community pharmacy (2 years), hospital pharmacy (4 years);
* Continued education (CE) and Continuous postgraduate development (CPD).

MASTER: complex skills in context
* Testing of knowledge, skills and behaviour is fully integrated (contextual) in courses;
* Increased attention for authentic tasks (patient care, medication policy, compounding), role-playing (patient interviews) and serious gaming (e.g. GIMMICS);
* Blended learning: clerkships in community pharmacy, hospital pharmacy and/or industry;
* Research project (individual).

BACHELOR: skills in isolation
* Assessment of knowledge is tested in individual tests (midterm, final) and group work (papers, project results) in the context of courses;
* Skills (calculations, compounding, laboratory skills, oral and written communication, management, ...) are tested or assessed in the context of courses, but ....
* If skills are assessed as 'insufficient' individual additional training and re-testing of separate skills is offered in the skills lab.

Figure 4. Example of curriculum layers for assessment of skills. Assessment formats in the curriculum ideally should move from simple, isolated assessments to more integrated, complex assessment formats. In this example the assessment principles of the pharmacy curriculum in Utrecht, including subsequent postgraduate education, are given as an example.

Several assessment formats have been developed for formative assessment in competency-based education, such as serious games [40], and tools for self-evaluation and reflection, such as portfolios [46,47]. Objective structured clinical examinations (OSCEs, [48]) and an internet-based assessment tool for the assessment of advanced pharmacy practice experiences [18] can be used for summative assessment. It is beyond the scope of this article to fully evaluate the range of available assessment tools and their use in CBPE (but see [22] for a recent overview of the issues involved).

- **Tip 6: Less is more, in particular for summative assessment.** A pharmacy curriculum is easily overburdened; this can lead to burnout of students and teachers. Restrict contact hours and high-stakes examinations to a well-chosen minimum; concentrate on non-summative feedback.
- **Tip 7: Use authentic assessment tasks.** Authentic learning activities and assessment tasks (cases, OSCE), simulations (serious gaming) and the use of entrustable professional activities (EPAs) can motivate students and can prepare them for their professional life.

7. Effective Learning and Constructive Alignment

Competency-based education heavily relies on constructivist psychological principles, in which educational methods focus on the learning of students [27,49,50], where students construct meaning from what they do during their learning activities. In step 5 of the curriculum design process (Figure 1), the role of the teachers is to design the teaching-learning environment (TLE) in such a way that the student cannot escape from learning. In order to reach this goal all aspects of the TLE needs to be carefully designed. The learning of students is not only influenced by their perception of the assessment tasks (see above), but also by the way teaching is delivered, by the teacher behavior, and by the rules and regulations which pertain to the curriculum. The principles of *constructive alignment* [27,31,51] can be used to align all aspects of the TLE as good as possible. Several examples of carefully designed pharmacy curricula are described in the literature (see Table 1).

It is recommended to use an explicit, evidence-based, educational model to guide the development of learning tasks and design principles for a curriculum (see Table 2 for an example). Once formulated, the model can be used to make argued choices for teaching and learning activities, assessment of students and organizational aspects, whenever discussions arise during the actual implementation of the curriculum. Having an explicit model for the learning process will also protect against taking potentially counterproductive measures (see [27], pp. 309–315).

Effective TLEs with high-quality learning outcomes need to be designed in such a way that students are motivated for deep, self-regulated, learning [31,44,52]. Several aspects of a model for effective learning are summarized in Figure 5. Extensive educational research has shown that—in addition to cognitive capacity—personality characteristics, motivational aspects, and teacher behaviors can contribute to the quality of learning [27,52]. Autonomous motivation, in contrast to controlled motivation, can contribute to high-quality outcomes [52,53]. As explained by the self-determination theory, student motivation is enhanced by giving students *autonomy* in studying and by creating opportunities to develop *relatedness* to fellow students and teachers, in addition to paying attention to the development of *competence* [52]. Problem- and/or project-based learning are educational methods, which are well-aligned with the development of the autonomy, relatedness and competence elements of this educational model [27,31]. Designing challenging student tasks and explicit attention for *reflection on learning* also will enhance the quality of learning outcomes. Case-based learning, for example, can be very effective for studying pharmacotherapy-oriented tasks and for practicing patient- and physician-directed communication. It is beyond the scope of this paper to describe all aspects of designing effective TLEs; excellent literature sources are available [12,27,51,52].

A newly-developed curriculum is seldom ideal from the start [54], and several years may be necessary to improve upon the original design. As a final step of the curriculum design process (Step 6 in Figure 1) a cycle of curriculum evaluation and refinement is needed. Both short-term and long-term feedback loops are necessary. In the short-term feedback loop all curricular elements (e.g., courses) are evaluated on a regular, usually annual, basis. In the long-term feedback loop the curriculum is undergoing review every five to ten years. This review may be synchronized with external evaluations or visitations, but is preferably also done internally.

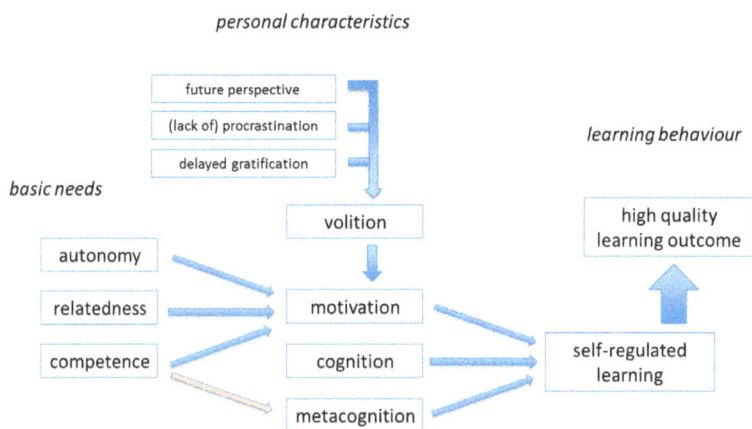

Figure 5. A model for effective learning.

Evaluation of the curriculum *as a whole* is usually done by mapping the curriculum using an existing framework [42,55]. Curriculum mapping can serve different purposes, but in the context of this paper the main purpose will be providing guidance in further improvement of the curriculum, as described by Farris et al. [30] and Zelenitsky et al. [56]. Mapping the *experienced curriculum* (the curriculum as perceived by the students) on the *intended curriculum* (the designed curriculum) can be very useful for identifying gaps, overlaps, and discontinuities in the curriculum construction [55,57].

- **Tip 8: Adopt frameworks for cognitive and skills development.** An explicit, evidence-based, educational model can guide choices for assessments, learning tasks, and can protect against counterproductive measures.
- **Tip 9: Use curriculum mapping for internal quality enhancement.** Mapping the various curricular elements (course, etc.) against existing frameworks can be very helpful in identifying curricular gaps, overlaps, and discontinuities.

8. Management and Quality Enhancement

When a new curriculum is designed, a continuous process of refinement and optimization is started. This is a long-term and laborious process, which may last several years [30,54] and requires an effective quality management system [58]. It is advised that continuity for this process is organized at the highest possible organizational level (faculty, institute) and that the adopted design principles (Section 5) and an explicit educational model (Section 7) are used as an internal 'frame of reference' to guide all discussions with the involved teachers, students, and other stakeholders. Open-minded and frequent communication with everybody involved is necessary to prevent misalignment of curricular elements and to assure that the delivered curriculum (the curriculum as presented to the students) is as close as possible to the designed curriculum. It is advised to use evaluation- and feedback-cycles at both the course level and the curriculum level (see above) to maintain flexibility and adaptability [58].

Integration of curricular disciplinary content, integration of knowledge and skills, and the use of novel assessment formats require that some teachers are given the opportunity to pay attention to these aspects of the curriculum, preferably on a curriculum level (i.e., under direct responsibility of a director of education or a curriculum manager). In this way the consistency of educational approaches in different curricular elements (across courses) can be improved. Appointment of stream coordinators, skills consultants, or specialization of teachers in novel assessment methodology is called for [59]. Another potential new teacher role is the role of a tutor, who can advise students in their personal development. All these non-traditional roles are preferably organized as temporary part-time tasks besides a primary role as teacher, responsible for delivering disciplinary content in the curriculum. By organizing non-traditional roles in this way, the connection with other teachers and flexibility of the organization can be maintained as good as possible. We strongly advise against a strict separation between teachers having traditional and non-traditional roles in the organization of the curriculum.

New roles for teachers require development of new educational expertise and the introduction of a trajectory for continuous professional development *as a teacher* [60]. This can be organized in a more or less structured way, ranging from formal training in teaching methodology [59], to a personal development trajectory for future program leaders [61,62]. Suggestions for the collaborative development of specific expertise can be found in the educational literature [63]. Depending on the local situation (such as size of a faculty or institution, number of teachers involved, existing university policy) educational development programs can range from informal, small-scale initiatives to relatively large-scale formal training and development programs [64]. Engaging in a scholarly approach to teaching and learning (SoTL), involving reflection on teaching experiences, use of educational research literature, and evidence-based development of teaching, can contribute to the quality enhancement of CBPE [65,66]. In our experience, the content and scale of training or development activities should be carefully adapted or 'titrated' to the needs felt by teachers [59,65]. Effective development programs usually involve a combination of individual and collaborative projects, sharing of knowledge and experiences, interaction with other like-minded teachers, and goal-directed development of educational innovations [61,64].

- **Tip 10: Assure management continuity.** Development and optimization of CBPE requires a long-term perspective and continuity in the educational development. This is best achieved by appointing a director of education and/or by forming a curriculum management team.
- **Tip 11: Develop educational expertise and specialization.** A competency-based curriculum requires teachers to develop expertise in the fields of autonomy-supportive teaching and competency assessment.
- **Tip 12: Develop scholarship of teaching and learning (SoTL).** Building a competence-based curriculum requires the development and testing of non-standard teaching-learning activities and novel assessment formats. Teachers and curriculum developers can benefit from a scholarly approach, using educational literature, exchange of good practices and training or coaching in (inter)national networks.

9. Summary and Conclusions

Implementing CBPE is a time-consuming and complicated process, which requires 'translation' of formulated competencies into intended learning outcomes and assessment formats. Conscious choices and decisions on all organizational levels are needed to achieve consistency between learning tasks, feedback to students, teacher roles, and organization of the curriculum. Formulating design principles and adopting an explicit educational model, based on evidence-based educational psychology, can be helpful in guiding curriculum development and optimization. Finally, the institutional management structure should support the required human resources allocation, which involves training of teachers for new roles and the stimulation of teacher professional development.

Acknowledgments: The authors to thank Antonio Sánchez Pozo (University of Granada, Spain), Aukje Mantel-Teeuwisse (Utrecht University, The Netherlands), and Daisy Volmer (Institute for Pharmacy, Tartu, Estonia) for commenting on an early version of this paper.

Author Contributions: Since 2000 the authors have been actively involved in developing competency-based curricula for undergraduate pharmacy (Andries Koster and Tom Schalekamp) and pharmaceutical sciences (Irma Meijerman) degrees. Andries Koster conceived the paper and wrote the first version; Tom Schalekamp and Irma Meijerman commented on several draft versions of the paper.

Conflicts of Interest: The authors declare no conflict of interest.

Appendix A. Competency- or Outcome-Based Frameworks

AACP 2013. CAPE Educational outcomes, American Association of Faculties of Pharmacy (AACP), Chicago 2013. Available online at www.aacp.org/resources/education/cape/Pages/default. aspx (last accessed on 8 February 2017).

AFPC 2010. Educational Outcomes for First Professional Degree Programs in Pharmacy (Entry to Practice Pharmacy Programs) in Canada. Association of Faculties of Pharmacy of Canada (AFPC), Vancouver 2010. Available online at http://www.afpc.info/node/39 (last accessed on 8 February 2017).

EPCF 2016. European Pharmacy Competency Framework, The Phar-QA Quality in Pharmacy Education in Europe consortium and European Association of Faculties of Pharmacy (EAFP), Brussels and Malta 2016. Available online at eec-pet.eu/pharmacy-education/competency-framework/ (last accessed on 8 February 2017).

FIP 2012. A global framework for services provided by Pharmacy workforce. International Pharmaceutical Federation (FIP), The Hague, 2012. Available online at www.fip.org/files/fip/ PharmacyEducation/GbCF_v1.pdf (last accessed on 1 December 2016).

GPhC 2011. Standards for the initial education and training of pharmacists, General Pharmaceutical Council (GPhC), 2011. Available online at www.pharmacyregulation.org/sites/ default/files/GPhC_Future_Pharmacists.pdf (last accessed on 1 December 2016).

NCSF 2010. National Competency Standards Framework for Pharmacists in Australia, Pharmaceutical Society for Australia (PSA), 2010. Available online at www.psa.org.au/downloads/ standards/competency-standards-complete.pdf (last accessed on 1 December 2016).

References

1. Girot, E.A. Assessment of Competence in Clinical Practice—A Review of the Literature. *Nurse Educ. Today* **1993**, *13*, 83–90. [CrossRef]
2. Spielman, A.I.; Fulmer, T.; Eisenberg, E.S.; Alfano, M.C. Dentistry, Nursing, and Medicine: A Comparison of Core Competencies. *J. Dent. Educ.* **2005**, *69*, 1257–1271. [PubMed]
3. Frank, J.R.; Snell, L.S.; Cate, O.T.; Holmboe, E.S.; Carraccio, C.; Swing, S.R.; Harris, P.; Glasgow, N.J.; Campbell, C.; Dath, D.; et al. Competency-Based Medical Education: Theory to Practice. *Med. Teach.* **2010**, *32*, 638–645. [CrossRef] [PubMed]
4. Bruno, A.; Bates, I.; Brock, T.; Anderson, C. Towards a Global Competency Framework. *Am. J. Pharm. Educ.* **2010**, *74*, 56. [CrossRef] [PubMed]
5. Nash, R.E.; Chalmers, L.; Brown, N.; Jackson, S.; Peterson, G. An International Review of the use of Competency Standards in Undergraduate Pharmacy Education. *Pharm. Educ.* **2015**, *15*, 131–141.
6. Hepler, C.D. Clinical Pharmacy, Pharmaceutical Care, and the Quality of Drug Therapy. *Pharmacotherapy* **2004**, *24*, 1491–1498. [CrossRef] [PubMed]
7. Miller, B.M.; Moore, D.E.; Stead, W.W.; Balser, J.R. Beyond Flexner: A New Model for Continuous Learning in the Health Professions. *Acad. Med.* **2010**, *85*, 266–272. [CrossRef] [PubMed]
8. Van Mil, J.W.F.; Schulz, M.; Tromp, T.F.J. Pharmaceutical Care, European Developments in Concepts, Implementation, Teaching, and Research: A Review. *Pharm. World Sci.* **2004**, *26*, 303–311. [PubMed]
9. Atkinson, J.; De Paepe, K.; Sanchez Pozo, A.; Rekkas, D.; Volmer, D.; Hirvonen, J.; Bozic, B.; Skowron, A.; Mirciou, C.; Marcincal, A.; et al. The Second Round of the Phar-QA Survey of Competences for Pharmacy Practice. *Pharmacy* **2016**, *4*, 27. [CrossRef]
10. Medina, M.S.; Plaza, C.M.; Stowe, C.D.; Robinson, E.T.; DeLander, G.; Beck, D.E.; Melchert, R.B.; Supernaw, R.B.; Roche, V.F.; Gleason, B.L.; et al. Center for the Advancement of Pharmacy Education 2013 Educational Outcomes. *Am. J. Pharm. Educ.* **2013**, *77*, 162. [CrossRef] [PubMed]
11. Pearson, M.L.; Hubball, H.T. Curricular Integration in Pharmacy Education. *Am. J. Pharm. Educ.* **2012**, *76*, 204. [CrossRef] [PubMed]
12. Meijerman, I.; Nab, J.; Koster, A.S. Designing and Implementing an Inquiry-Based Undergraduate Curriculum in Pharmaceutical Sciences. *Curr. Pharm. Teach. Learn.* **2016**, *8*, 905–919. [CrossRef]

13. Koster, A.S.; Meijerman, I.; Blom, L.T.G.; Schalekamp, T. Pharmacy Education at Utrecht University: An Educational Continuum. *Dosis Sci. J. Pharm.* **2009**, *25*, 85–93.
14. Gibbs, G.; Knapper, C.; Piccinin, S. Disciplinary and Contextually Appropriate Approaches to Leadership of Teaching in Research-Intensive Academic Departments in Higher Education. *High. Educ. Q.* **2008**, *62*, 416–436. [CrossRef]
15. Stupans, I.; McAllister, S.; Clifford, R.; Hughes, J.; Krass, I.; March, G.; Owen, S.; Woulfe, J. Nationwide Collaborative Development of Learning Outcomes and Exemplar Standards for Australian Pharmacy Programmes. *Int. J. Pharm. Pract.* **2015**, *23*, 283–291. [CrossRef] [PubMed]
16. Miller, G.E. The Assessment of Clinical Skills/Competence/Performance. *Acad. Med.* **1990**, *65*, S63–S67. [CrossRef] [PubMed]
17. Stupans, I.; Atkinson, J.; Mestrovic, A.; Nash, R.; Rouse, M.J. A Shared Focus: Comparing the Australian, Canadian, United Kingdom and United States Pharmacy Learning Outcome Frameworks and the Global Competency Framework. *Pharmacy* **2016**, *4*, 26. [CrossRef]
18. Ried, L.D.; Doty, R.E.; Nemire, R.E. A Psychometric Evaluation of an Advanced Pharmacy Practice Experience Clinical Competency Framework. *Am. J. Pharm. Educ.* **2015**, *79*, 19. [CrossRef] [PubMed]
19. Ramia, E.; Salameh, P.; Btaiche, I.F.; Saad, A.H. Mapping and Assessment of Personal and Professional Development Skills in a Pharmacy Curriculum. *BMC Med. Educ.* **2016**, *16*, 533. [CrossRef] [PubMed]
20. Midlöv, P.; Höglund, P.; Eriksson, T.; Diehl, A.; Edgren, G. Developing a Competency-Based Curriculum in Basic and Clinical Pharmacology—A Delphi Study among Physicians. *Basic Clin. Pharm. Toxicol.* **2015**, *117*, 413–420. [CrossRef] [PubMed]
21. Silva, H.; Stonier, P.; Buhler, F.; Deslypere, J.-P.; Criscuolo, D.; Nell, G.; Massud, J.; Geary, S.; Schenk, J.; Kerpel-Fronius, S.; et al. Core Competencies for Pharmaceutical Physicians and Drug Development Scientists. *Front. Pharm.* **2013**, *4*, 105. [CrossRef] [PubMed]
22. Hawkins, R.E.; Welcher, C.M.; Holmboe, E.S.; Kirk, L.M.; Norcini, J.J.; Simons, K.B.; Skochelak, S.E. Implementation of Competency-Based Medical Education: Are We Addressing the Concerns and Challenges? *Med. Educ.* **2015**, *49*, 1086–1102. [CrossRef] [PubMed]
23. Ten Cate, O.; Scheele, F. Viewpoint: Competency-Based Postgraduate Training: Can We Bridge the Gap between Theory and Clinical Practice? *Acad. Med.* **2007**, *82*, 542–547. [CrossRef] [PubMed]
24. Chen, H.C.; van den Broek, W.E.S.; Ten Cate, O. The Case for use of Entrustable Professional Activities in Undergraduate Medical Education. *Acad. Med.* **2015**, *90*, 431–436. [CrossRef] [PubMed]
25. Pittenger, A.L.; Chapman, S.A.; Frail, C.K.; Moon, J.Y.; Undeberg, M.R.; Orzoff, J.H. Entrustable Professional Activities for Pharmacy Practice. *Am. J. Pharm. Educ.* **2016**, *80*, 57. [CrossRef] [PubMed]
26. Buurma, H.J. *Advanced Community Pharmacist Education Programme*; Royal Dutch Pharmacists Association: The Hague, The Netherlands, 2012.
27. Biggs, J.; Tang, C. *Teaching for Quality Learning at University*, 4th ed.; SRHE and Open University Press, McGraw-Hill: Maidenhead, UK, 2011.
28. Harden, R.M. Learning Outcomes as a Tool to Assess Progression. *Med. Teach.* **2007**, *29*, 678–682. [CrossRef] [PubMed]
29. Al-Eraky, M.M. Curriculum Navigator: Aspiring Towards a Comprehensive Package for Curriculum Planning. *Med. Teach.* **2012**, *34*, 724–732. [CrossRef] [PubMed]
30. Farris, K.B.; Demb, A.; Janke, K.K.; Kelley, K.; Scott, S.A. Assessment to Transform Competency-Based Curricula. *Am. J. Pharm. Educ.* **2009**, *73*, 158. [CrossRef] [PubMed]
31. Katajavuori, N.; Hakkarainen, K.; Kuosa, T.; Airaksinen, M.; Hirvonen, J.; Holm, Y. Curriculum Reform in Finnish Pharmacy Education. *Am. J. Pharm. Educ.* **2009**, *73*, 151. [CrossRef] [PubMed]
32. Boyce, E.G.; Lawson, L.A. Preprofessional Curriculum in Preparation for Doctor of Pharmacy Educational Programs. *Am. J. Pharm. Educ.* **2009**, *73*, 155. [CrossRef] [PubMed]
33. Ho, S.S.S.; Kember, D.; Lau, C.B.S.; Au Yeung, M.Y.M.; Leung, D.Y.P.; Chow, M.S.S. An Outcomes-Based Approach to Curriculum Development in Pharmacy. *Am. J. Pharm. Educ.* **2009**, *73*, 14. [CrossRef] [PubMed]
34. Nelson, M.; Allison, S.D.; McCollum, M.; Luckey, S.W.; Clark, D.R.; Paulsen, S.M.; Malhotra, J.; Brunner, L.J. The Regis Model for Pharmacy Education: A Highly Integrated Curriculum Delivered by Team-Based Learning™ (TBL). *Curr. Pharm. Teach. Learn.* **2013**, *5*, 555–563. [CrossRef]

35. Poloyac, S.M.; Empey, K.M.; Rohan, L.C.; Skledar, S.J.; Empey, P.E.; Nolin, T.D.; Bies, R.R.; Gibbs, R.B.; Folan, M.; Kroboth, P.D. Core Competencies for Research Training in the Clinical Pharmaceutical Sciences. *Am. J. Pharm. Educ.* **2011**, *75*, 27. [CrossRef] [PubMed]

36. Newble, D.; Stark, P.; Bax, N.; Lawson, M. Developing an Outcome-Focused Core Curriculum. *Med. Educ.* **2005**, *39*, 680–687. [CrossRef] [PubMed]

37. Mak-Van Der Vossen, M.; Peerdeman, S.; Kleinveld, J.; Kusurkar, R. How We Designed and Implemented Teaching, Training, and Assessment of Professional Behaviour at VUmc School of Medical Sciences Amsterdam. *Med. Teach.* **2013**, *35*, 709–714. [CrossRef] [PubMed]

38. Mulder, H.; Cate, O.T.; Daalder, R.; Berkvens, J. Building a Competency-Based Workplace Curriculum around Entrustable Professional Activities: The Case of Physician Assistant Training. *Med. Teach.* **2010**, *32*, e453–e459. [CrossRef] [PubMed]

39. Husband, A.K.; Todd, A.; Fulton, J. Integrating Science and Practice in Pharmacy Curricula. *Am. J. Pharm. Educ.* **2014**, *78*, 63. [CrossRef] [PubMed]

40. Van der Werf, J.J.; Dekens-Konter, J.; Brouwers, J.R.B.J. A New Model for Teaching Pharmaceutical Care Services Management. *Pharm. Educ.* **2004**, *4*, 165–169. [CrossRef]

41. Conway, S.E.; Medina, M.S.; Letassy, N.A.; Britton, M.L. Assessment of Streams of Knowledge, Skill, and Attitude Development across the Doctor of Pharmacy Curriculum. *Am. J. Pharm. Educ.* **2011**, *75*, 83. [CrossRef] [PubMed]

42. Malone, D.T.; Short, J.L.; Naidu, S.; White, P.J.; Kirkpatrick, C.M. Mapping of the Australian Qualifications Framework Standards Onto an Undergraduate Bachelor of Pharmacy Course. *Pharm. Educ.* **2015**, *15*, 261–269.

43. Van Der Vleuten, C.P.M.; Schuwirth, L.W.T.; Driessen, E.W.; Dijkstra, J.; Tigelaar, D.; Baartman, L.K.J.; van Tartwijk, J. A Model for Programmatic Assessment Fit for Purpose. *Med. Teach.* **2012**, *34*, 205–214. [CrossRef] [PubMed]

44. Nicol, D.; MacFarlane-Dick, D. Formative Assessment and Selfregulated Learning: A Model and Seven Principles of Good Feedback Practice. *Stud. High. Educ.* **2006**, *31*, 199–218. [CrossRef]

45. Schuwirth, L.W.T.; Van der Vleuten, C.P.M. Programmatic Assessment: From Assessment of Learning to Assessment for Learning. *Med. Teach.* **2011**, *33*, 478–485. [CrossRef] [PubMed]

46. Stupans, I.; March, G.; Owen, S.M. Enhancing Learning in Clinical Placements: Reflective Practice, Self-Assessment, Rubrics and Scaffolding. *Assess. Eval. High. Educ.* **2013**, *38*, 507–519. [CrossRef]

47. Allen, S.; Waterfield, J.; Rivers, P. An Investigation of Pharmacy Student Perception of Competence-Based Learning using the Individual Skills Evaluation and Development Program, iSED®. *Pharm. Educ.* **2016**, *16*, 72–80.

48. Branch, C. An Assessment of Students' Performance and Satisfaction with an OSCE Early in an Undergraduate Pharmacy Curriculum. *Curr. Pharm. Teach. Learn.* **2014**, *6*, 22–31. [CrossRef]

49. Ten Cate, O.; Snell, L.; Mann, K.; Vermunt, J. Orienting Teaching toward the Learning Process. *Acad. Med.* **2004**, *79*, 219–228. [CrossRef] [PubMed]

50. Blumberg, P. Maximizing Learning through Course Alignment and Experience with Different Types of Knowledge. *Innov. High. Educ.* **2009**, *34*, 93–103. [CrossRef]

51. Kaartinen-Koutaniemi, M.; Katajavuori, N. Enhancing the Development of Pharmacy Education by Changing Pharmacy Teaching. *Pharm. Educ.* **2006**, *6*, 197–208. [CrossRef]

52. Ten Cate, T.J.; Kusurkar, R.A.; Williams, G.C. How Self-Determination Theory can Assist our Understanding of the Teaching and Learning Processes in Medical Education. *AMEE Guide No. 59. Med. Teach.* **2011**, *33*, 961–973. [PubMed]

53. Niemiec, C.P.; Ryan, R.M. Autonomy, Competence, and Relatedness in the Classroom: Applying Self-Determination Theory to Educational Practice. *Theor. Res. Educ.* **2009**, *7*, 133–144. [CrossRef]

54. Remington, T.L.; Hershock, C.; Klein, K.C.; Niemer, R.K.; Bleske, B.E. Lessons from the Trenches: Implementing Team-Based Learning Across several Courses. *Curr. Pharm. Teach. Learn.* **2015**, *7*, 121–130. [CrossRef]

55. Plaza, C.M.; Draugalis, J.R.; Slack, M.K.; Skrepnek, G.H.; Sauer, K.A. Curriculum Mapping in Program Assessment and Evaluation. *Am. J. Pharm. Educ.* **2007**, *71*, 20. [CrossRef] [PubMed]

56. Zelenitsky, S.; Vercaigne, L.; Davies, N.M.; Davis, C.; Renaud, R.; Kristjanson, C. Using Curriculum Mapping to Engage Faculty Members in the Analysis of a Pharmacy Program. *Am. J. Pharm. Educ.* **2014**, *78*, 139. [CrossRef] [PubMed]

57. Kirkpatrick, M.A.F.; Pugh, C.B. Assessment of Curricular Competency Outcomes. *Am. J. Pharm. Educ.* **2001**, *65*, 217–224.

58. Kleijnen, J.; Dolmans, D.; Willems, J.; van Hout, H. Effective Quality Management Requires a Systematic Approach and a Flexible Organisational Culture: A Qualitative Study among Academic Staff. *Q. High Educ.* **2014**, *20*, 103–126. [CrossRef]

59. Andurkar, S.; Fjortoft, N.; Sincak, C.; Todd, T. Development of a Center for Teaching Excellence. *Am. J. Pharm. Educ.* **2010**, *74*, 123. [CrossRef] [PubMed]

60. Al-Eraky, M.M.; Donkers, J.; Wajid, G.; Van Merrienboer, J.J.G. Faculty Development for Learning and Teaching of Medical Professionalism. *Med. Teach.* **2015**, *37*, S40–S46. [CrossRef] [PubMed]

61. Tofade, T.; Abate, M.; Fu, Y. Perceptions of a Continuing Professional Development Portfolio Model to Enhance the Scholarship of Teaching and Learning. *J. Pharm. Pract.* **2014**, *27*, 131–137. [CrossRef] [PubMed]

62. Grunefeld, H.; van Tartwijk, J.; Jongen, H.; Wubbels, T. Design and Effects of an Academic Development Programme on Leadership for Educational Change. *Int. J. Acad. Dev.* **2015**, *20*, 306–318. [CrossRef]

63. Vos, S.S.; Trewet, C.B. A Comprehensive Approach to Preceptor Development. *Am. J. Pharm. Educ.* **2012**, *76*, 47. [CrossRef] [PubMed]

64. Mårtensson, K.; Roxå, T.; Olsson, T. Developing a Quality Culture through the Scholarship of Teaching and Learning. *High. Educ. Res. Dev.* **2011**, *30*, 51–62. [CrossRef]

65. Medina, M.; Hammer, D.; Rose, R.; Scott, S.; Creekmore, F.M.; Pittenger, A.; Soltis, R.; Bouldin, A.; Schwarz, L.; Piascik, P. Demonstrating Excellence in Pharmacy Teaching through Scholarship. *Curr. Pharm. Teach. Learn.* **2011**, *3*, 255–259. [CrossRef]

66. Dolmans, D.H.J.M.; Tigelaar, D. Building Bridges between Theory and Practice in Medical Education using a Design-Based Research Approach: AMEE Guide No. 60. *Med. Teach.* **2012**, *34*, 1–10. [CrossRef] [PubMed]

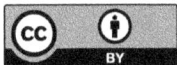

pharmacy

MDPI

Article

How Two Small Pharmacy Schools' Competency Standards Compare with an International Competency Framework and How Well These Schools Prepare Students for International Placements

John Hawboldt [1], Rose Nash [2] and Beverly FitzPatrick [1,*]

[1]   School of Pharmacy, Memorial University, St. John's, NL A1B3V6, Canada; hawboldt@mun.ca
[2]   Public Health and Global Health, School of Medicine, University of Tasmania, Hobart 7000, Australia; rose.mcshane@utas.edu.au
*   Correspondence: bfitzpatrick@mun.ca; Tel.: +1-709-777-2407

Academic Editor: Jeffrey Atkinson
Received: 4 February 2017; Accepted: 28 February 2017; Published: 6 March 2017

Abstract: International standards of pharmacy curricula are necessary to ensure student readiness for international placements. This paper explores whether curricula from two pharmacy programs, in Australia and Canada, are congruent with international standards and if students feel prepared for international placements. Nationally prescribed educational standards for the two schools were compared to each other and then against the International Pharmaceutical Federation (FIP) Global Competency Framework. Written student reflections complemented this analysis. Mapping results suggested substantial agreement between the FIP framework and Australia and Canada, with two gaps being identified. Moreover, the students felt their programs prepared them for their international placements. Despite differences in countries, pharmacy programs, and health-systems all students acclimatized to their new practice sites. Implications are that if pharmacy programs align well with FIP, pharmacists should be able to integrate and practise in other jurisdictions that also align with the FIP. This has implications for the mobility of pharmacy practitioners to countries not of their origin of training.

Keywords: international placement; pharmacy undergraduates; curriculum; standards

1. Introduction

Pharmacy education, in the era of globalization, should consider international practice experience placements (PEP) for pharmacy students. International PEP can increase students' cultural competence, enhance awareness of other health-systems, and provide exposure to diseases/medicines that may be uncommon in their respective countries. Alsharif indicated that international experiences can increase students' respect for local, national, international, and ethnic identities [1]. Moreover, Cisneros et al., suggested that these placements can also increase students' contributions to global healthcare [2]. Through PEP, Owen argued that students are provided with situations that enhance the knowledge and teaching gained through classic university education as they are immersed in real patient-care settings under the supervision of professional practitioners [3]. International placements should be useful as they can assist in the preparation of future pharmacists for the challenges of a multicultural and increasingly globalized world.

Students enrolled in Pharmacy courses at The University of Tasmania, Australia (UTas) and Memorial University, Newfoundland and Labrador, Canada (MUN) request varied placement experiences and sites that offer diverse community and institutional health experiences. This includes interdisciplinary involvement, patient-centred care, quality sites, experienced preceptors, and travel opportunities. Currently, UTas and MUN have a reciprocal arrangement that offers opportunities for students to complete PEP in Australia and Canada.

The schools are located in different parts of the world, one in the southeast hemisphere, and the other in the northwest hemisphere. Both are on islands, rather than the mainland of each country. Thus, there are social, demographic and geographical similarities, as well as different challenges. UTas was established in 1890, and the Pharmacy School in 1978. MUN opened in 1925, and the School of Pharmacy in 1985. By international standards, the schools are relatively young and face challenges associated with market demands and shifting workplace expectations.

Both populations have an identifiable founder population with little immigration as compared to other states or provinces. In Tasmania, approximately 90% of its people are born in Australia and are primarily of British descent [4]. Tasmania has two major centres of population (Hobart and Launceston) on opposite side of the Island. Newfoundland started with about 20,000 settlers in 1760 with approximately 98% of the current population being of English or Irish descent [5] Newfoundland also has two major population centres (The Avalon Peninsula and the city of Corner Brook) again, also on opposites sides of the Island. Anecdotally, the three authors of this article would agree that there is also a form of discrimination against both Island populations from their mainland counterparts in the forms of jokes about their respective genetic profiles or with regards to perceived levels of intelligence. All of these factors, including a historical "Island induced" social isolation from their mainland countrymen, has led to many similarities between both Tasmania and Newfoundland.

In terms of health care, in Australia the government provides subsidised healthcare and medicines through Medicare and the Pharmaceutical Benefits Scheme in Hospitals and the Community setting. Medicare is partially funded by income tax surcharges. While Australians enjoy free public hospital services, all patients make "means tested contributions" to their other healthcare and medication costs. Individuals can get private health cover to increase their choices, get access to services, and receive subsidised care on "private services". In Canada, there is a single payer (the provincial Government) when it comes to medicines delivered in the institutional setting. However, in the community setting, medicines may be provided by a private insurer (with or without a co-pay), exclusively by the provincial government, partially by the provincial government (with a co-pay), or the patient pays out-of-pocket.

With regards to educational programs, the Australians provide a "degree plus professional registration" while the Canadian pharmacy programs follow a "registration upon graduation" system. A main difference between these two programs is that the majority of practice experience is provided to the Australian students after they graduate from their program under the guidance of a preceptor and intern training provider; while in Canadian programs, the practice experiences are integrated within the program at least once per academic year.

Students in UTas are able to enter their pharmacy program straight out of high school and graduate from a four year program with a Bachelor of Pharmacy. Students at MUN require a minimum one year of university with specific credits and graduate from a four year pharmacy program with a Bachelor of Science in Pharmacy. Both UTas and MUN students have raised concerns about the quality of their local placement sites, the practices they are observing, and the alignment of practice with their university studies and personal expectations. The fact that this is occurring in both schools speaks to similarities found in both programs and also supports the argument that pharmacy education around the world has more similarities than differences.

Medicine was one of the first health-care professions to attempt to develop a global competency framework, the purpose being to ensure that competencies for all physicians, despite geographic area, will be transparent, applicable, and transferable to other jurisdictions [6]. Regardless of socioeconomic, cultural, teaching, and health-systems differences between countries, the World Federation for Medical Education believes that the basic science of medicine is universal [6]. The International Pharmaceutical Federation (FIP), advocates a similar position for Pharmacy Education [6]. Thus, FIP developed the Global Competency Framework (GCF) as a mapping tool that deals with initial education and training for those who have an interest in globalizing or harmonizing the expectations of what a pharmacy practitioner should be [6]. The GCF was developed from an extensive literature review on pharmacy competencies and practice with a comparative study that identified common behaviors that should be applicable to the pharmacy workforce worldwide [6]. The GCF was intended to be used as a mapping tool that would evolve with the profession. The document consisted of four domains (e.g., pharmaceutical public health—a population focus), various competencies (e.g., health promotion) and behaviors associated with each competency [6]. This was done with the intent of providing outcomes in the training and practice of pharmacists. This in turn would therefore be useful to regulators and educators who are interested in promoting global consistency with regards to the expectation of practice for pharmacy practitioners [6].

In order for an international PEP to be effective, the educational experiences of the PEP must align with the respective programs' expectations and learning objectives. Moreover, FIP has acknowledged, "Practitioner Development frameworks, containing a structured assembly of behavioral competencies have become increasingly popular in professional education, driven by the need for transparency in the training, development and professional recognition of healthcare professionals" [6] (p. 3). Our research questions are twofold: how comparable are the respective Australian and Canadian competencies with the FIP Framework, and how well prepared do the students from the two schools feel to complete their international placements.

2. Materials and Methods

To establish how well students from UTas and MUN are prepared for global pharmacy practice, we used two methods of data collection. To answer the first research question, we analysed the curriculum standards associated with each program. This was achieved by mapping the educational outcomes from both pharmacy schools against the GCF of FIP [6]. For the mapping in this study, the FIP GCF was used as a common denominator as it sets a global pharmacy standard to which the educational outcomes could be compared. Each outcome from the Australian and Canadian documents, and then the FIP GCF, was analysed for content and meaning to determine if there were matching outcomes in the documents. The individual authors from each respective country completed mapping of country specific educational outcomes with FIP. Then, the authors from both countries worked together to find the commonalities and differences between their countries, and with FIP. This involved several meetings through Skype to achieve common understandings of the outcomes and to reach consensus on the mapping. As well, numerous emails transpired between the authors on an ongoing basis throughout the analysis.

The educational outcome documents from Australia and Canada included: the Australian Pharmacy (AP) Threshold Learning Outcomes (PhLOs), the National Competency Standards (NCSs) Framework for Pharmacists in Australia (PA), The Association of Faculties of Pharmacy of Canada (AFPC) Educational Outcomes (EOs) for First Professional Degree Programs in Pharmacy in Canada, and the National Association of Pharmacy Regulatory Authorities (NAPRA) Professional Competencies (PCs) for Canadian Pharmacists at Entry to Practice [3,7–9]. Although each school has course objectives which are mapped against each school's national competencies, this level of analysis was not included in this paper. Because this mapping had already been conducted, the authors were confident that the national outcome documents reflected the goals and outcomes for their individual schools. Thus, mapping was done at the national level for the purpose of this paper.

To address the second research question we went directly to students who were participating in an international PEP. This allowed a more complete understanding of the meaning of the outcomes and how they related to international standards, as it gave us a student perspective of what they were learning. Four students from UTas and two students from MUN participated in an international PEP, where they spent six weeks in each other's Schools. The students had completed three years of their programs before the placements. We endeavoured to learn what the students experienced in their programs and how they used this knowledge in their international PEP.

As part of the PEP the students wrote reflections, based on specific guidelines developed by one of the authors who has experience in education and qualitative research, about the commonalities and differences they observed and experienced during their placements, how this related to the education they received in their pharmacy programs, and whether they thought they were prepared to practise globally. See Table 1 for reflection guidelines. These data were first cycle structurally coded for concepts to examine commonalities, differences, and relationships, and then second cycle pattern coded to search for major themes and explanations in the data [10]. First cycle coding is the initial coding where broad categories are developed and second cycle coding follows to more fine tune the categories and develop specific concepts. We used structural coding for the initial analysis which examined how the students answered the questions and to establish a framework for the results. In our second cycle of coding we looked for patterns to develop themes and explanations. Ethics as per the Helsinki declaration was obtained for all participants.

Table 1. Guidelines for Student Reflections.

Write about the SPE in the second country and relate it to the pharmacy program you received in your own country. Include how well the pharmacy program in your country prepared you for the SPE in the second country. Suggested guidelines are below. Please add anything else that comes to mind, including examples of specific incidences.
Write about: • Similarities   • Differences   • What was easy in the second country   • What was difficult in the second country   • What it was (specifically) in your program that made it possible/practicable for you to do a SPE in a second country   • The most important learning(s) you got from your program   • The most important learning(s) in the second country   • What you learned during the SPE that was new and that you might not be able to put into practice in your own country

3. Results

3.1. Mapping Results

The top-level domains of each document are listed in Table 2. Where possible, mapping proceeded to the furthest sub-domain in each document.

Table 2. Top Level Domains of the Australian Pharmacy (AP) Threshold Learning Outcomes (PhLOs) and CSs, the Canadian Association of Faculties of Pharmacy of Canada (AFPC) EDs and National Association of Pharmacy Regulatory Authorities, Professional Competencies (NAPRA PCs), and the International Pharmaceutical Federation, Global Competency Framework (FIP GCF) [3,6–9].

Jurisdictions	Top-Level Domains
Australian Pharmacy Threshold Learning Outcomes	1. "Demonstrate professional behaviour and accountability in the commitment to care for and about people". 2. "Retrieve, critically evaluate, and apply evidence in professional practice". 3. "Demonstrate team and leadership skills to deliver safe and effective practice". 4. "Make, act on, and take responsibility for clinically, ethically, and scientifically sound decisions". 5. "Communicate in lay and professional language, choosing strategies appropriate for the context and diverse audiences". 6. "Reflect on current skills, knowledge, attitudes, and practice; planning and implementing for ongoing personal and professional development". 7. "Apply pharmaceutical, medication, and health knowledge and skills: -Within their scope of practice, in the assessment of individual health status and medication needs, and where necessary, develop, implement and monitor management plans in consultation with patients/clients and other health professionals to improve patient outcomes, and -To promote and optimise the health and welfare of communities and/or populations". 8. "Formulate, prepare, and also supply medications and therapeutic products".

Table 2. *Cont.*

Jurisdictions	Top-Level Domains
National Competency Standards Framework for Pharmacists in Australia	Domain 1: "Professional and ethical practice addressing the legal, ethical and professional responsibilities of pharmacists". Domain 2: "Communication, collaboration, and self-management required to communicate effectively with consumers and colleagues, and build and maintain cooperative working relationships within the healthcare team". Domain 3: "Leadership and management relating to how pharmacists apply management and organisational skills ensuring the effective and efficient delivery of pharmacy services". Domain 4: "Review and supply prescribed medicines for accurate and timely supply of prescription medicines, including extemporaneously prepared products". Domain 5: "Prepare pharmaceutical products required for the extemporaneous preparation of single or multiple units of a medicine for immediate issue and/or use by a specific consumer". Domain 6: "Deliver primary and preventative health care addressing the role pharmacists have in encouraging and assisting individual and groups of consumers to take responsibility for their own health". Domain 7: "Promote and contribute to optimal use of medicines addressing aspects of clinical practice directed that ensures the safe and appropriate management of medicines". Domain 8: "Critical analysis, research, and education addressing the capability of pharmacists to analyse and synthesise information from medical and pharmaceutical literature".
Association of Faculties of Pharmacy of Canada Educational Outcomes for First Professional Degree Programs in Pharmacy in Canada,	Care Provider: "Pharmacy graduates use their knowledge, skills, and professional judgement to provide pharmaceutical care and manage a patient's medication and overall health needs". Communicator: "Pharmacy graduates communicate with diverse audiences, using various strategies that consider the situation, intended outcomes of the communication, and the target audience". Collaborator: "Pharmacy graduates work collaboratively with teams to provide effective health care and to fulfil their professional obligations to the community at large". Manager: "Pharmacy graduates use management skills to optimize patient care ensuring the safe and effective distribution of medications, and efficient use of health resources". Advocate: "Pharmacy graduates advance the health and well-being of individual patients, communities, and populations, and support pharmacists' professional roles". Scholar: "Pharmacy graduates apply the knowledge and skills required to be a medication therapy expert, and are able to master, generate, interpret, and disseminate pharmaceutical and pharmacy practice knowledge". Professional: "Pharmacy graduates honour their roles as self-regulated professionals through both individual patient care and fulfilment of their professional obligations to the profession, and the community".
National Association of Pharmacy Regulatory Authorities Professional Competencies (PCs) for Canadian Pharmacists at Entry to Practice	Ethical, Legal and Professional Responsibilities: "Pharmacists practise within legal requirements, demonstrate professionalism, and uphold professional standards of practice, codes of ethics, and policies". Patient Care: "Pharmacists, in partnership with the patient and in collaboration with other health professionals, meet the patient's health and drug-related needs to achieve the patient's health goals". Product Distribution: "Pharmacists ensure accurate product distribution that is safe and appropriate for the patient". Practice Setting: "Pharmacists oversee the practice setting with the goal of ensuring safe, effective and efficient patient care". Health Promotion: "Pharmacists use their expertise to advance the health and wellness of patients, communities and populations". Knowledge and Research Application: "Pharmacists access, retrieve, critically analyse and apply relevant information to make evidence-informed decisions ensuring safe and effective patient care". Communication and Education: "Pharmacists communicate effectively with patients, the pharmacy team, other health professionals, and the public, providing education when required". Intra and Inter-Professional Collaboration: "Pharmacists work in collaboration with the pharmacy team and other health professionals to deliver comprehensive services, make best use of resources, and ensure continuity of care in order to achieve the patient's health goals". Quality and Safety: "Pharmacists collaborate in developing, implementing, and evaluating policies, procedures, and activities that promote quality and safety".
International Pharmaceutical Federation Global Competency Framework	1. "Pharmaceutical Public Health Competencies where the pharmacist will be involved in such activities as health promotion and medicines information/advice". 2. "Pharmaceutical Care Competencies whereby pharmacists will assess effective use of medicines, compound medicines, dispense medicines, monitor medicine therapy, and provide patient consultation/diagnosis". 3. "Organization and Management Competencies where concepts such as budget/reimbursement, human resources management, improvement of service, procurement, supply chain, supply management and work place management are provided". 4. "Professional/Personal Competencies where pharmacists will apply concepts such as communication skill improvement, the importance of continuing professional development, legal/regulatory practice, professional/ethical practice, quality assurance/research in the workplace and self management".

After the mapping was completed, only two gaps were evident. First, AFPC did not map against FIP or any of the Australian documents regarding compounding of medicines. The specific FIP competency missed included:

"Prepare pharmaceutical medicines (e.g., extemporaneous, cytotoxic medicines), determine the requirements for preparation (calculations, appropriate formulation, procedures, raw materials, equipment etc.).

Compound under the good manufacturing practice for pharmaceutical (GMP) medicines."

The second gap was in the FIP domain of organization and management competencies. This was again exclusively with one competency document, the AP PhLOs. The gap determined was in:

"Acknowledge the organizational structure.

Effectively set and apply budgets.

Ensure appropriate claim for reimbursement.

Ensure financial transparency.

Ensure proper reference sources for service reimbursement."

Other than these two gaps, the mapping revealed consistency across all domains in all of the documents. Moreover, these particular gaps were not evident with the NCS and NAPRA documents. Most importantly, improving patient care was a consistent theme present in all competencies.

3.2. Student Reflections

The students thought that similar topics were taught in both programs, but the emphases placed on specific concepts within these topics differed in the two schools. For example, while both groups of students studied therapeutics, the students from UTas thought the MUN students spent more time learning about medications and their effects on patients than the patient being the centre of care. One student stated that MUN had a drug-oriented approach with "goals of care for each single medication", whereas UTas had a patient oriented approach with "goals of care for the patient as a whole". The UTas students thought MUN was more academically focused on facts and theory, while the Utas program concentrated more on practical outcomes such as patient interaction, critical thinking, and communication skills. Instructors from both Schools discussed the student comments and considered them as teaching and learning points for future instruction.

Students from both schools participate in experiential learning during their programs, and all students thought there were similar expectations from the preceptors in both countries. MUN students participate in experiential placements each year of their program, some of which are six weeks in duration. UTas students have fewer and shorter placements, but participate in fortnightly hospital visits where they are encouraged to interact with actual patients. Students from both countries discussed advantages and disadvantages of the different types of experiential learning. For example, one student from UTas thought that "at the end of three weeks a student may just be feeling comfortable, then they are moved to the next placement", but at MUN with the six-week placement, students get the opportunity to "become better accustomed to the workplace". In both countries, students reported that medication reconciliation is important and made the observation that they observed mutual respect between pharmacists and physicians.

All the students thought they were adequately prepared to complete their PEP. They had to get used to different drugs and brand names, and some differences in what constituted controlled substances. Students also had to learn about the different healthcare systems in each country. However, the differences between the two countries were not surmountable. One student said it this way, "the programs are similar in what we learn, especially therapeutically, this enabled me to apply that knowledge here and effectively work as I would have at home, with the same expectations".

4. Discussion

There was strong agreement regarding standards and competencies among the documents. The Australian (PhLOs and NCS) and Canadian (AFPC and NAPRA) standards aligned strongly with the FIP standards, and aligned well with each other. The PhLOs and AFPC EOs did not match the FIP GCF with respect to two particular "practical" competencies, those being compounding and management principles. This is despite the fact that these principles are provided in both curricula and are everyday activities of practising pharmacies. These competencies were covered by the respective documents (NAPRA PCs and NCS for AP), which primarily deal with the practice component of a pharmacist's training.

The strong agreement among the respective documents is also reflected in the students' written reflections. With the exception of a few key points, such as patient-focus versus patient–drug focus, and some regulatory issues, all the students appeared to integrate well into the individual practice experience. This was evident from the positive student and preceptor comments. Further, no students or their respective preceptors identified adjustment issues, even though both countries have slightly different health-systems and pharmacy programs. Despite these health-system differences, the students accommodated to their new practice sites with minimal discomfort. In addition, the students' ability to practise effectively in another jurisdiction was not affected by the differences between the two programs in how and when students participate in their experiential learning.

There are reasons beyond the mapping and student reflections that could contribute to the ease with which these students completed their PEP. Possibilities include language (both are primarily English speaking locations), ethno-cultural similarities (both have highly homogenized, traditionally Anglo-Saxon populations), and although slightly different, the health-systems are still first world, and would have a high degree of similarity in the services they provide.

Limitations of this paper include the small sample size for the student reflections, but the student comments should be used judiciously for generalization. They provide an example of student experiences in international placements that are not meant to be universal, but complement the document analysis to provide context and meaning to our comparison.

Since this positive experience, the MUN School of Pharmacy has increased its intake of international students to include students from Australia and the United States. Moreover, MUN students continue to participate in PEP in Australia and are now in other countries such as the United States. UTas continues to send student to MUN and elsewhere. Both schools see the value in the internationalization of their practice experiences in that not only do the students see how another healthcare system provides for its citizens, they also are exposed to the unique role that the pharmacists play in that system. It is these learnings that they can take back to their respective jurisdictions and act as agents of change.

5. Conclusions

Despite differences in countries, pharmacy programs, and health-systems the students from both countries successfully completed their international practice experience placements at their new practice sites. This is encouraging as it implies that if the standards and competencies of pharmacy programs have good alignment with the international standards of GCF, then PEP will not be affected by the differences in students' education at individual schools. Moreover, this has implications for the mobility of pharmacy practitioners to countries not of their origin of training. More research needs to be conducted to determine if these findings would apply to practising pharmacists who might like to transition to other countries.

Author Contributions: John Hawboldt, Rose Nash and Beverly FitzPatrick conceived and designed the paper; John Hawboldt and Rose Nash aligned the stated competencies/outcomes; John Hawboldt, Rose Nash, Beverly FitzPatrick wrote the paper.

Conflicts of Interest: The authors declare no conflict of interest.

Pharmacy **2017**, *5*, 14

References

1. Alsharif, N.Z. Globalization of Pharmacy Education: What is Needed? *Am. J. Pharm. Educ.* **2012**, *76*, 77. [CrossRef] [PubMed]
2. Cisneros, R.M.; Jawaid, S.P.; Kendall, D.A.; Mcpherson, C.E.; Mu, K.; Weston, G.C.; Roberts, K.B. International Practice Experiences in Pharmacy Education. *Am. J. Pharm. Educ.* **2013**, *77*, 188. [CrossRef] [PubMed]
3. Stupans, I.; McAllister, S.M.; Clifford, R.; Hughes, J.; Krass, I.; March, G.; Owen, S.; Woulfe, J. Nationwide collaborative development of learning outcomes and exemplar standards for Australian pharmacy programs. *Int. J. Pharm. Pract.* **2014**, *23*, 283–291. [CrossRef] [PubMed]
4. Scott, P.; Roe, S. Tasmania. Encyclopaedia Britannica. Available online: https://www.britannica.com/place/Tasmania (accessed on 21 February 2017).
5. Rahman, P.; Jones, A.; Curtis, J.; Bartlett, S.; Peddle, L.; Fernandez, B.; Freimer, N. The Newfoundland population: A unique resource for genetic investigation of complex diseases. *Hum. Mol. Genet.* **2004**, *13*, 167–172. [CrossRef]
6. The International Pharmaceutical Federation. FIP Education Initiatives: Pharmacy Education Taskforce A Global Competency Framework. 2012. Available online: https://www.fip.org/files/fip/PharmacyEducation/GbCF_v1.pdf (accessed on 25 January 2017).
7. Pharmaceutical Society of Australia. National Competency Standards Framework for Pharmacists in Australia. 2010. Available online: http://www.psa.org.au/supporting-practice/national-competency-standards (accessed on 25 January 2017).
8. Association of Faculties of Pharmacy in Canada. Educational Outcomes for First Professional Degree Programs in Pharmacy (Entry-to-Practice Pharmacy Programs) in Canada. Available online: https://www.afpc.info/sites/default/files/AFPC%20Educational%20Outcomes.pdf (accessed on 25 January 2017).
9. National Association of Pharmacy Regulatory Authorities. National Association of Pharmacy Regulatory Authorities: Professional Competencies (PCs) for Canadian Pharmacists at Entry to Practice. 2014. Available online: http://napra.ca/Content_Files/Files/Comp_for_Cdn_PHARMACISTS_at_EntrytoPractice_March2014_b.pdf (accessed on 25 January 2017).
10. Saldana, J. *The Coding Manual for Qualitative Researchers*, 2nd ed.; Sage Publications: Thousand Oaks, CA, USA, 2013; pp. 84–86 and 207–213.

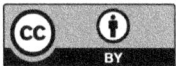

pharmacy

MDPI

Article

CPD Aligned to Competency Standards to Support Quality Practice

Rose Nash [1,*], Wendy Thompson [2,3], Ieva Stupans [4], Esther T. L. Lau [2],
Jose Manuel Serrano Santos [2], Natalie Brown [5], Lisa M. Nissen [2,3] and Leanne Chalmers [1]

[1] School of Medicine, University of Tasmania, Private Bag 34, Hobart, TAS 7000, Australia;
leanne.chalmers@utas.edu.au

[2] School of Clinical Sciences, Queensland University of Technology, 2 George St., Brisbane, QLD 4000,
Australia; wendy.thompson@qut.edu.au (W.T.); et.lau@qut.edu.au (E.T.L.L.);
manuel.serranosantos@qut.edu.au (J.M.S.S.); l.nissen@qut.edu.au (L.M.N.)

[3] School of Pharmacy, University of Queensland, Brisbane, QLD 4102, Australia

[4] School of Health and Biomedical Sciences, RMIT University, P.O. Box 71, Bundoora, VIC 3083, Australia;
ieva.stupans@rmit.edu.au

[5] Tasmanian Institute of Learning and Teaching, University of Tasmania, Sandy Bay, TAS 7005, Australia;
natalie.brown@utas.edu.au

* Correspondence: Rose.McShane@utas.edu.au; Tel.: +61-400-341-758

Academic Editor: Jeffrey Atkinson
Received: 30 December 2016; Accepted: 20 February 2017; Published: 25 February 2017

Abstract: As medication experts, pharmacists are key members of the patient's healthcare team. Pharmacists must maintain their competence to practice to remain responsive to the increasingly complex healthcare sector. This paper seeks to determine how competence training for pharmacists may enhance quality in their professional development. Results of two separately administered surveys (2012 and 2013) were compared to examine the reported continued professional development (CPD) practices of Australian pharmacists. Examination of results from both studies enabled a focus on how the competency standards inform CPD practice. In the survey administered in 2012, 91% ($n = 253/278$) pharmacists reported that they knew their current registration requirements. However, in the survey administered in 2013, only 43% ($n = 46/107$) reported utilization of the National Competency Standards Framework for Pharmacists in Australia (NCS) to self-asses their practice as part of their annual re-registration requirements. Fewer, 23% ($n = 25/107$), used the NCS to plan their CPD. This may be symptomatic of poor familiarity with the NCS, uncertainty around undertaking self-directed learning as part of a structured learning plan and/or misunderstandings around what CPD should include. This is supported by thematic analysis of pharmacists' social media comments. Initial and ongoing competence training to support meaningful CPD requires urgent attention in Australia. The competence (knowledge, skills and attributes) required to engage in meaningful CPD practice should be introduced and developed prior to entry into practice; other countries may find they are in a similar position.

Keywords: competency; continued professional development; lifelong learning

1. Introduction

As health professionals, the public holds pharmacists accountable for maintaining their knowledge, skills and attributes (competence) to practice with each personal interaction—be it at the hospital bedside, in a community pharmacy, general practice (general practice provides person centred, continuing, comprehensive and coordinated whole-person health care to individuals and families in their communities (accessed on 13 January 2017 at http://www.racgp.org.au/becomingagp/what-is-a-gp/what-is-general-practice/)) clinic or when administering a vaccination. This accountability directly translates to patient safety. For most health professionals competence, practice and Continued Professional Development (CPD) are inseparable. Competence has many definitions and meanings in the literature [1]. The Australian Pharmacy profession defines it as follows:

'Competence to mean that an individual possesses the required knowledge, skills and attributes sufficient to successfully and consistently perform a specific function or task to a desired standard ... Inherent to the concept of competence is the inference of assessment of performance in a given circumstance against a specified external measure.' [2] (pp. 4–5)

For Australian pharmacists this external measure is the National Competency Standards Framework for Pharmacists in Australia (NCS) [2] and the Professional Practice Standards [3], as shown in Table 1.

Table 1. National Competency Standards Framework (2010) and Professional Practice Standards (2010) for Australian Pharmacists [2,3].

National Competency Standards Framework
1. Professional and Ethical Practice
2. Communication, Collaboration and self-management
3. Leadership and Management
4. Review and supply prescribed medicines
5. Prepare pharmaceutical products
6. Deliver primary and preventative health care
7. Promote and contribute to optimal use of medicines
8. Critical analysis, research and education
Professional Practice Standards
1. Fundamental Pharmacy Practice
2. Managing Pharmacy Practice
3. Counselling
4. Medication Review
5. Dispensing
6. Indirect Pharmacy Services
7. Dose Administration Aids Service
8. Services to Residential Care Facilities
9. Continuity of Care through Medication Liaison Services
10. Compounding (also known as Extemporaneous Dispensing)
11. Compounding Sterile Preparations
12. Provision of Non-prescription Medicines and Therapeutic Devices
13. Health Promotion
14. Medicines Information Centres
15. Pharmacy services to Aboriginal and Torres Strait Islander Health Services
16. Screening and Risk Assessment
17. Disease State Management
18. Harm Minimisation

The National Safety and Quality Health Service Standards, 2012 describe competency-based training as *'an approach to training that places emphasis on what a person can do in the workplace as a result of training completion'* [4] (p. 8). For Australian pharmacists this 'training' would usually include university studies with experiential placements, a supervised internship and an individual's ongoing CPD. In this paper the authors have intentionally separated competency-based training into two elements: skills development for lifelong learning and the overall competence of the individual to practice. Whilst it is recognized that the skills for lifelong learning are essential to the maintenance of one's competence, this paper will be focused on the competence-based training required for meaningful lifelong learning.

As described elsewhere in the literature, lifelong learning and CPD are often considered interchangeable terms [5–8]. Jane Ryan [5] interviewed nurses, physiotherapists (physical therapists) and occupational therapists to explore their understanding of lifelong learning. Their responses were themed around continuous learning, reflection, reflective practice, personal and/or professional development. Their responses reinforce why the literature often describes lifelong learning and CPD interchangeably. In the pharmacy profession, Rouse has described CPD as a framework for lifelong learning [6].

Currently most health professionals, including pharmacists, self-regulate their competence to practice, thus the attributes (motivation, honesty, morals, ethical consciousness, professionalism) and skills (self-assessment, reflection, informed judgment, critical appraisal) developed pre-career will inform the quality and safety of their future practice. Professionals from other health disciplines report their motivation for participating in CPD as updating their professional knowledge, updating existing qualifications, increasing the status of the profession as a whole and demonstrating individual professional competence [5].

Traditional Continued Education (CE) delivery has been described by Konstantinides as *'material presented in an online or live classroom format. The learning consists of listening and reading, then applying the information to an assessment, often in the form of a multiple-choice exam.'* He states that, in contrast, CPD *'asks more of the pharmacist.'* [9] (p. 2). As discussed by Konstantinides, the American Institute of Medicine [10] identified an urgent need to reform the continuing education (CE) system in 2009, citing concern regarding poorly constructed vision, a lack of inter-professional approach to education delivery, and general concerns about regulation and evaluation of continuing education [9]. In recognition that health knowledge has an increasingly short half-life [11], ongoing learning must be targeted to support the competence of the individual in their context. Expanding scopes of practice and uncertainty around the definition and exact skills of the health professional of the future reinforce the importance and need for competence informed CPD practice. Reassuringly, the importance of lifelong learning has been highlighted by the international pharmacy community for some time, as one of the essential elements of the Eight Star Pharmacist [12].

In 2010, the Pharmacy Board of Australia (PBA) introduced the CPD framework. For Australian pharmacists CPD is currently classified into three sub-groups;

- **Group 1** (one CPD credit per hour of activity): information accessed without assessment (e.g., didactic presentations, and activities with little or no attendee interaction).
- **Group 2** (two CPD credits per hour of activity): knowledge or skills improved with assessment (e.g., activities where the participant's acquisition of knowledge or skills can be demonstrated).
- **Group 3** (three CPD credits per hour of activity): quality or practice-improvement facilitated (e.g., activities where an assessment of existing practice (of an individual or within a pharmacy practice), and the needs and barriers to changes in this practice, is undertaken prior to the development of a particular activity. As a result, the activity addresses identified professional development needs with a reflection post-activity to evaluate practice change or outcomes resulting from the activity. Such an activity will most likely extend over a number of weeks or months [13].

Pharmacists in Australia must evidence 40 points of CPD each year (consisting of no more than 20 Group 1 points) [13]. A mandatory requirement, as outlined in the CPD standards, is that all Australian pharmacists must self-assess against the NCS to identify their individual learning needs. The Pharmacy Board of Australia describes CPD as *'the means by which members of the profession continue to maintain, improve and broaden their knowledge, expertise and competence, and develop the personal and professional qualities required throughout their professional lives'* [13].

In December 2015, the Pharmacy Board of Australia announced the requirement that all Australian pharmacists provide evidence of a learning plan. Based on the principles of Kolb's learning cycle [14] the Pharmacy Board of Australia CPD framework consists of five steps. **Plan**: In considering their professional role and services provided, pharmacists are to identify and document professional development opportunities. **Do**: Pharmacists then carry out a range of activities related to their scope of practice and professional development needs. **Record**: A record of CPD activities is to be made and kept for three full CPD cycles. **Reflect**: Pharmacists must consider how the activities have impacted their practice. **Incorporate**: Pharmacists then must ensure the insight and learning from CPD is actively incorporated into future practice. These steps are described in Figure 1.

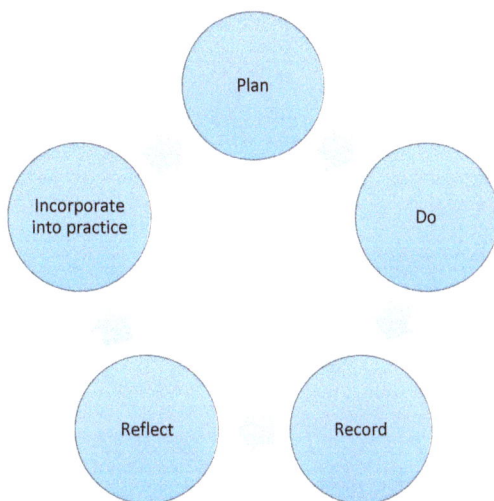

Figure 1. The Pharmacy Board of Australia CPD plan/record framework [15].

Given this context, it is clear that to ensure patient safety and quality service provision and to support the advanced practice aims of the pharmacy profession, educators need to replace passive knowledge transfer approaches with self-directed learning approaches. In particular, educators must support pharmacy students, with developing skills and attributes alongside and interwoven with the requisite expert knowledge. On the whole, higher education appears to have accepted this challenge, evidenced in the move towards outcomes-focused learning rather than the traditional input-based model, which traditionally focused on an indicative curriculum [16–18]. In the medical profession outcomes-based education has been accepted since the 1990s [17]. The dialogue from accreditation agencies including the Tertiary Education Quality Standards Agency and professional bodies such as the Australian Pharmacy Council [19] also endorses this approach to learning. In addition, the recent emphasis on work-integrated learning [20,21], project-based assessment [22], portfolio assessment [23–25] and 'authentic assessment' strategies [26] give confidence in our ability to support graduates from all disciplines to succeed in the 'real world'. This approach to learning and assessment can better provide pharmacy graduates with the necessary skills and attributes to survive the continual change and complexity inherent in our health system. Of relevance, this complexity is predicted to increase.

As previously highlighted by Fernandez et al. not all educators support the movement towards competency based education, and their arguments deserve mention [27]. Given the importance of these issues to the Australian Pharmacy profession, this research sought to determine:

1. How Australian pharmacists understand the CPD framework;
2. How their CPD is being guided by the NCS;
3. Whether pharmacists employ best practice strategies in their Professional Development;
4. What education models can improve the quality of CPD practice in the future.

2. Materials and Methods

2.1. Methodology

The study utilised a pragmatist frame and concurrent strategy of enquiry [28]. Consistent with this research approach, two separate surveys were administered online; each captured quantitative data around the understanding and use of the CPD framework, demonstrating multiple viewpoints from the profession. In addition, Survey 2 also captured qualitative responses, further exploring these views. Whilst anecdotal, the social media response to the Board's announcement of CPD plans provides an interesting narrative. These findings were triangulated to explore the use and understanding of the Australian CPD requirements for greater meaning. Triangulation of *'data sources is a means for seeking convergence across qualitative and quantitative methods'* [28] (p. 15).

2.2. Method

2.2.1. Survey 1. How Is the CPD Framework Understood by Pharmacists?

WT worked in collaboration with the PBA, who reviewed the questions and advised on the content of the questionnaire. The online survey was piloted with a small group of practicing pharmacists and adjusted and amended accordingly before disseminating (September 2012 to end of October 2012). Links were made available in newsletters of the Pharmaceutical Society of Australia (PSA), the Society of Hospital Pharmacists of Australia (SHPA), and the PBA. To increase the response rate, a paper-based version was also disseminated in September 2012 to pharmacists attending two different CPD seminars in Brisbane, hosted by the SHPA and PSA, respectively. The sampling technique employed was non-probability sampling [29] and targeted Australian Registered Pharmacists. Responses were summarised using descriptive statistics. Ethics approval was granted by the University of Queensland's Human Research Ethics Committee (2012000467). For a full list of survey questions refer to Appendix A.

2.2.2. Survey 2. Current Knowledge, Use and Acceptance of the NCS by Australian Pharmacists

This online survey was open from November 2013 to June 2014 and invited all Australian students, interns, educators and registered pharmacists to participate. The sampling technique combined snowball and convenience sampling [30] and was disseminated using a combination of social media and conference presentation. As described in greater detail elsewhere [31], participants that were interviewed for a related project were also invited to distribute the survey to their networks via email. Qualitative responses were analysed using thematic analysis [32]. Quantitative responses were analysed using non-parametric techniques in SPSS V22 software (IBM: Armonk, NY, USA, 2013). Minimal risk ethics approval was obtained from the Tasmanian Social Sciences Human Research Ethics Committee (H13591). For a full list of survey questions refer to Appendix B.

2.2.3. Social Media Comments Posted on Australian Pharmacist Forums

Independently, RN and IS searched commonly accessed social media forums for pharmacists for comments on CPD plans. The comments made by pharmacists on board requirements to complete a CPD plan were identified by RN and IS and combined and duplicates removed. Search terms utilised included; CPD plan, Pharmacy and Australia. The dates were intentionally restricted to August 2016 to coincide with the media releases by the PBA and the week leading up to the end of the CPD cycle. The comments were analysed independently by three authors (IS, MS, NB) using thematic analysis techniques [32]. Emergent themes were discussed for consensus and are reported in Figure 3. All comments are provided in Appendix C.

3. Results

3.1. Response Rate

3.1.1. Survey 1. How Is the CPD Framework Understood by Pharmacists?

A total of 278 registered pharmacists responded to the survey representing approximately 1% of registered Australian pharmacists ($n = 25,944$). All responses were included, even though some were only partially completed [33,34].

3.1.2. Survey 2. Current Knowledge, Use and Acceptance of the NCS by Australian Pharmacists

Of the 660 online survey responses, 413 were full responses and 247 were incomplete; 527 participants (who responded to five or more questions) were included. Whilst the original survey invited provisional (intern) pharmacists, educators, students and registered pharmacists, only the responses from registered pharmacists (including preceptors who are by definition registered pharmacists) will be reported on here. The results from all respondents are reported elsewhere [31]. This sample ($n = 158$) represented less than 1% of registered Australian pharmacists.

3.1.3. Social Media Comments Posted on Australian Pharmacist Forums

The social media comments from a sub-section of the Australian pharmacist population (totalling 55 comments) were harvested from the most commonly accessed professional pharmacy forums (Pharmacy news, AJP.com.au). These comments were posted on four separate forums between 22 and 29 August 2016.

3.2. Participant Demographics

In Survey 1, respondents' ages ranged from 20 to 65+ years, with all 10 age brackets represented and age distribution correlated to the national pharmacy census data reported by Australian Health Practitioner Regulation Agency (AHPRA) in 2011 [33]. Sixty-six percent were female, 30% were male and 4% did not disclose their gender. Fifty-six percent of respondents had been on the Australian pharmacist register (after their intern year) for more than 10 years, 16% for six to 10 years, 24% for up to five years and 4% unknown. Fifty-four percent of participants identified their primary area of practice as community pharmacy, 27% were primarily practising as hospital pharmacists, and the remaining 19% were split across a number of sectors, e.g., pharmaceutical industry, consultancy or academia. Demographics of survey respondents for Survey 2 are summarised in Table 2.

Table 2. Participant demographics for Survey 2.

	Pharmacist ~
Completed survey	128
Incomplete survey	56
	158
State (workplace) ($n = 151$)	
TAS	49
NSW	25
QLD	37
Other	40
Professional Organisation aligned ($n = 158$) **	
PSA	110
SHPA	26
Guild	54
Other	104

Table 2. *Cont.*

	Pharmacist ˜
Member of Professional Organisation offers accredited CPD (*n* = 158)	
Yes	145
Area of Practice (*n* = 158) **	
Academia	3
Hospital	20
Community	125
Accredited	34
Other	18
Currently Practising (*n* = 158) [a]	
Yes	153
Years Practice (*n* = 156)	
1–5 years	47
5–10 years	30
10–15 years	18
15–30 years	34
30 years plus	27
Hours per week paid/actual (*n* = 153)	
1–10 h	6
10–30 h	32
30–40 h	64
40 h plus	51

Changes in denominator (*n*) are due to some respondents answering some questions and not others. ˜ Pharmacist includes pharmacists and preceptors. ** Pharmacists could select more than one category in answering some questions. [a] Currently practicing by Australian Health Practitioner Regulation Agency (AHPRA) definition. *States*: TAS—Tasmania, NSW—New South Wales, QLD—Queensland, Other—Northern Territory, Australian Capital Territory, Victoria, Western Australia, South Australia. *Organisation*: PSA—Pharmaceutical Society of Australia, SHPA—Society of Hospital Pharmacists of Australia, Guild—Pharmacy Guild of Australia. *Other areas of practice*: Drug & Alcohol Services, Practice Support, Administration role, Prison Service, Clinical Services, Government, Education (National Prescribing Service Facilitator), Unemployed, Rural, General Practitioner, Committee Member, Pharmaceutical Industry.

3.3. Survey Results

3.3.1. Survey 1

The majority of respondents were accepting of the CPD framework and felt they understood the requirements. These findings have been reported in greater detail elsewhere [34]. However, when more specific questions were asked to discern their understanding of the CPD framework and its intended use, it was clear that there were gaps in the responding pharmacists' knowledge (Table 3).

Table 3. Survey 1. How is the CPD framework understood by pharmacists?

Statements	% Agreement
1. I know the current CPD requirements for general registration.	91% (*n* = 253/278)
2. There has been enough guidance on CPD requirements.	77% (*n* = 215/278)
3. I know how to undertake self-directed learning as part of a structured learning plan.	57% (*n* = 158/278)
4. CPD is also known as continuing education.	76% (*n* = 210/278)

3.3.2. Survey 2

Overall, despite many pharmacists confirming knowledge of the NCS [31], pharmacists' familiarity with the profession's NCS was found to be sub-optimal (Table 4). Just over half of the responding pharmacists reported that they did not use the NCS for renewal of annual registration (57%, 61/107). The majority confirmed they did not use the NCS when planning their CPD (77%, 82/107). Their barriers and suggested solutions to use of the NCS, as reported elsewhere [31], are provided in Figure 2.

Table 4. Survey 2. Pharmacists' current knowledge, use and acceptance of the NCS.

Statements	% Agreement
1. I know what the NCS are.	83% ($n = 115/139$)
2. I am not familiar (not at all/not very) with the NCS.	90% ($n = 120/134$)
3. I am familiar (familiar/very familiar/extremely familiar) with the NCS.	10% ($n = 14/134$)
4. I use the NCS for renewal of my annual registration.	43% ($n = 46/107$)
5. I use the NCS to plan my CPD.	23% ($n = 25/107$)

Whilst the details and sample comments from the participants are provided elsewhere [31], a summary of the themes that emerged from the thematic analysis is presented in Figure 2 below.

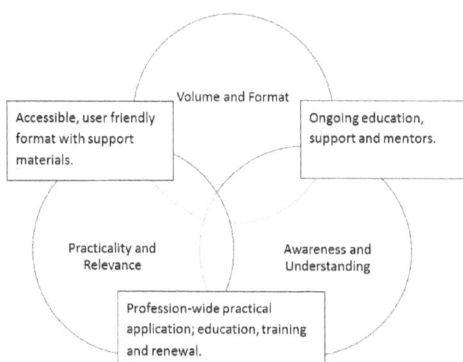

Figure 2. Themes derived from respondents reported barriers (circles) and enablers (rectangles) to use of NCS [31].

3.3.3. Social Media Comments

There was good consensus in the thematic analysis carried out by three independent authors, which led to the development of four clear themes, presented with their sub-themes in Figure 3.

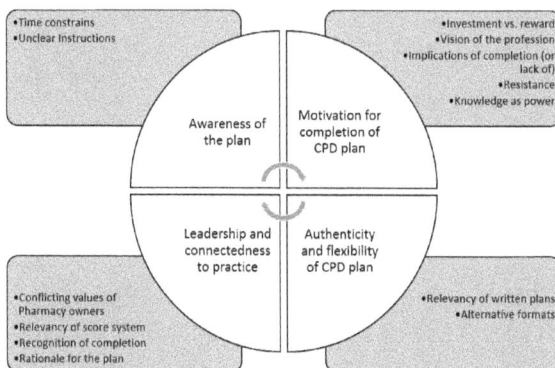

Figure 3. Themes derived from thematic analysis of social media comments.

3.3.4. Triangulation of All Three Sources

The major issues identified in the surveys included: "I know how to undertake self-directed learning as part of a structured learning plan" (Survey 1) with poor familiarity of the NCS and use of them to plan CPD (Survey 2). These issues align with the 'instructions', 'connectedness to practice' and 'relevance' sub-themes in the thematic analysis (Figure 3), which also provides additional depth around further issues. There is also some crossover in the themes from the social media comments and the qualitative aspect from Survey 2: for example, pharmacists questioning the relevance of CPD plans/NCS, concern regarding adequate awareness and understanding of each. Triangulation of the three sources highlights that respondent pharmacists want mentoring, support, education and clear instruction on the professions' expectations around CPD plans, lifelong learning and the use of NCS in the process.

4. Discussion

How can competence training enhance quality in professional development? Increasingly there is a recognition that universities are now responsible for facilitating a graduate's development of their knowledge, skills and attributes (competence). As evidence of this, the Australian Qualifications Framework [35] states that a graduate at bachelor's level and above will be responsible and accountable for their learning needs. One essential skill desirable for all health professionals, including pharmacists, is their ability to engage in lifelong learning. This requires appropriate CPD habit formation and the development of metacognitive strategies such as self-assessment, informed judgment and reflection on action [36]. The Australian Pharmacy Council requires Australian pharmacy courses to provide evidence that their courses align with the NCS [19]. Although this is the case, this may not always be explicit to the student [37].

4.1. Pharmacists

Our findings highlight that prior to the introduction of the compulsory CPD plan (December 2015) the respondent pharmacists' understanding and engagement with the CPD framework was not optimal. This sub-group of Australian pharmacists reported that they had failed to comply with the mandatory requirement set by the PBA to self-assess their practice against the NCS at their annual re-registration. They also did not appear to understand aspects of the CPD framework, as reflected in their perception on how CE (distinct pockets of learning) differed from CPD. At the time Survey 2 was administered (2013–2014), pharmacists appeared to be indicating that they were even less inclined to use the NCS to inform their CPD [34]. It is acknowledged that this finding preceded the December 2015 PBA announcement that the CPD plan/record framework would be a mandatory requirement for all Australian pharmacists. These findings highlight that some pharmacists may not appreciate the essential link between their practice, the NCS, CPD and the importance of tying all three together in meaningful CPD plans and active reflective learning cycles.

The 76% agreement that CE and CPD were equivalent in Survey 1 suggests CPD was just a number of CE events to get credits and that the pharmacists who responded did not appreciate the role of the intended learning cycle. In addition, Survey 2 suggests that the Australian pharmacists who responded were not using the NCS to assess their competency to practice despite this being mandated. The profession's suggested barriers and enablers (Figure 2) derived from the same survey data and reported elsewhere [31] help to explain why use of the NCS in CPD planning may have been sub-optimal. These barriers were reinforced by pharmacist comments on social media (August 2016) following the release of CPD plan requirements by the PBA.

Whilst anecdotal in nature, the 2016 responses on social media (Appendix C) highlight that some Australian pharmacists are not meaningfully engaging in CPD. These comments may provide insight into the survey results. For this sub-group of pharmacists who shared their 55 comments, CPD planning is perceived as burdensome, time-intensive, inconsistent with how and what they need to learn for their practice and an insult to them as a professional. Some commented that the PBA's requirement to develop a CPD plan is asking too much based on pharmacists' wages and is over and above other health professionals' CPD requirements. It is acknowledged that this sample may not represent the views of all Australian pharmacists and formal research is required to expand on this narrative further. Despite the small sample size, the results from this analysis are in alignment with those from the surveys and highlight views that are relevant to at least a part of the profession.

4.2. Education on NCS and Learning Cycle

These findings identified gaps in participating Australian pharmacists' knowledge on the competent use of the CPD framework, and align with issues recognized internationally in CPD practice. In a review of CPD practice in the United Kingdom, Donyai et al. described that the understanding of fundamental aspects of the CPD process appears to remain an issue in pharmacy. Examples of barriers to conducting CPD include the inability to distinguish between CE and CPD, difficulties in assessing one's own learning needs, and difficulty reflecting and evaluating one's learning [38]. This indicates that an optimal CPD process will require guidance and preparation, and questions whether pharmacy curriculum is currently providing enough guidance on its use. Curricula should be equipping Australian pharmacists to have a better understanding in these areas of the NCS and CPD framework, especially as there is clear evidence that engagement in self-regulated learning can result in better learning outcomes [39–41]. A pilot study carried out in the United States has identified that appropriate training and support can facilitate competence in the use of a CPD approach to lifelong learning and professional development. With guidance, study participants were using specific, measurable, achievable, relevant, and time-sensitive (SMART) objectives and developing a more structured learning plan with a specific timeline and outcomes in mind. They were confident in their planning and were able to pick activities that met their objectives, rather than just selecting the most convenient activity [42]. Introduction of an e-portfolio, which provides reference to the NCS and a structured approach to document learning and development, has the potential to be important in the development of pharmacists prior to registration. This tool facilitates a platform to direct the assessment of skills required and matches and records learning to the appropriate areas of NCS competence that is being developed. This guided approach could combat the issues that have been identified in the response to the CPD plan and those previously identified in the identification, documentation and inefficiency of pharmacists' CPD processes [38]. Providing clear instruction and increasing efficiency of the process may improve acceptance and usability.

To ensure a commitment to lifelong learning, the pharmacy curriculum must also emphasise the importance of CPD, especially as motivation to carry it out is not clear to some pharmacists (see themes identified in response to CPD plan). Assessment of their process in implementing a cycle of CPD planning could be one way of encouraging students to take the activity seriously, as it is widely recognised as a way of achieving student learning outcomes [41,43]. Formative assessment with feedback and summative assessment could provide students with the basic skills that will allow them to continue to learn and carry out CPD [41,43]. Educators should strive to emulate a motivation for learning and endeavour to share their CPD processes or skills. Additionally, as accreditation aims to produce graduates with the required knowledge and skills for internship, educators must consider whether enough guidance is being provided to our future pharmacists. It is not realistic to assume that Australian pharmacy students and even pharmacists have the requisite self-assessment skills to carry out CPD, given that international literature suggests students and registered pharmacists find self-assessment complex and challenging [44–46].

4.3. Limitations

Survey response rates were poor and likely represent more motivated individuals, resulting in selection bias. Whilst appropriate to the research questions and methodology chosen, the sampling techniques employed here (snowball, convenience and probability sampling) are likely to result in sampling bias, as are the low number of responses. The authors acknowledge the survey respondents may not represent the views of all Australian pharmacists. Similarly, the social media comments are a sub-sample and thus do not represent all Australian pharmacists. Whilst the social media forums are targeted at pharmacists, there is the potential for non-pharmacists to contribute to these forums given that they are publicly available. This research is specific to an Australian context, so potentially has limited transferability to an international audience.

4.4. Future Research

Future research should include longitudinal studies to explore the effect of early introduction (beginning of undergraduate studies) and meaningful use of the NCS, CPD (reflective cycles), and self-assessment on practitioner CPD practices. Investigation into whether learning plans informed by NCS correlate with pharmacist competence is required, as is a deeper understanding of what encourages competence and personal and professional development. Potentially useful to accreditation agencies is the identification of what motivates pharmacists to maintain competence and engage in lifelong learning, asking specifically if it is their job, peer pressure, patient centeredness, compliance attitudes or other motivators. Pharmacists could be surveyed to establish if the introduction of compulsory CPD plans in Australia in 2015 has improved their understanding and acceptance of CPD and led to increased use of the NCS in CPD practice. Larger-scale surveys with the pharmacy profession to further explore the themes identified from the social media analysis are required to confirm if the themes are representative of the general opinion of the profession on the implementation of CPD plans.

5. Conclusions

Currently some Australian pharmacists are not familiar with their NCS. Pharmacists also have limited understanding of the CPD framework. Of concern, a profession's mandatory requirements around self-regulation of competence are not always upheld in practice. Introduction of both elements (NCS and CPD Framework) earlier, during undergraduate studies, may translate to familiarity and more meaningful use through appropriate CPD habit formation. This is one example of how competence training may enhance quality in professional development. This finding may be applicable to all pharmacy educators internationally.

Acknowledgments: Wendy Thompson received a UQ New Staff Start up Grant (2011) to assist with work on Survey 1.

Author Contributions: Rose Nash and Wendy Thompson conceived and designed the paper; Rose Nash, Ieva Stupans, Leanne Chalmers, Natalie Brown, Wendy Thompson and Lisa M. Nissen administered the surveys; Rose Nash and Wendy Thompson analysed the survey data; Ieva Stupans, Jose Manuel Serrano Santos and Natalie Brown carried out thematic analysis of social media comments; Rose Nash, Wendy Thompson, Ieva Stupans, Jose Manuel Serrano Santos, Esther T. L. Lau, Lisa M. Nissen, Leanne Chalmers and Natalie Brown wrote the paper.

Conflicts of Interest: The authors declare no conflict of interest.

Appendix Survey 1 Questions

Dear Pharmacist,

The Pharmacy Board now requires registered pharmacists to acquire annual Continuing Professional Development (CPD) credits for renewal of registration. This online survey will aim to investigate what registered pharmacists understand about mandatory CPD by asking how you are managing to complete your annual CPD credits.

It would be appreciated and of considerable value if you could spend approximately 10 min completing this survey. Please note that the Pharmacy Board of Australia has provided the link to the survey to you on behalf of the UQ research team and names or contact details of participants will not be disclosed to the research team.

Participation in the survey is voluntary, but completing a survey will allow entry into a prize draw, which provides an opportunity to win a $50 Myers gift voucher.

If you would like to participate, then read the attached participant information leaflet (see the link at the end of question 1).This provides a more detailed explanation of what the study involves.

Participation in the survey will contribute to understanding how pharmacists are dealing with the introduction of mandatory CPD, and the resulting data may identify if further assistance or modifications could improve the process.

Thank you for considering this request.

Note: Continuing Professional Development will be referred to as CPD.

1. Before starting this survey, please can you confirm that you have read and understood the participant information leaflet and that you consent to participate in this survey? Click here for participant information.

- Yes, I have read the participant information and I agree to participate.
- No, I do not wish to participate.

To help us put your answers into context, please can you answer the following questions before you start the survey on CPD?

2. Approximately how long have you been on the register of pharmacists in Australia (after your intern year)?

- 0–5 years
- 6–10 years
- more than 10 years

3. What is your gender?

- Male
- Female

4. Please indicate your age bracket.

- 20–24 years
- 25–29 years
- 30–34 years
- 35–39 years
- 40–44 years
- 45–49 years
- 50–54 years
- 55–59 years
- 60–64 years
- 65 years or above

5. What is your main area of practice?

- Hospital
- Community
- Academia
- Not practising
- Consultants/accredited
- Other (please specify)

This page is just for practising Pharmacists.

6. Approximately how many hours per week do you work as a pharmacist?

- Part-time; 15 h or less
- Part-time; more than 15 h
- Fulltime

The questions on this page ask how you found out about mandatory CPD and investigate how well you understand the process.

7. Please show your level of agreement with the following statements. KEY: SA = Strongly Agree, A = Agree, N = Neutral, D = Disagree, SD = Strongly Disagree.

- I know the current CPD requirements for general registration.
- There has been enough guidance to outline the CPD requirements for renewal of registration.

8. Which source has provided the most information about the CPD requirements?

- Pharmacy Board of Australia
- Pharmaceutical Society of Australia
- Society of Hospital Pharmacists
- Pharmacy Guild
- Other (please specify)

The questions on this page will explore in more detail what you understand about the CPD process and ask which type of CPD you prefer.

9. The Pharmacy Board has classified CPD activities into three groups and each group acquires a different number of CPD credits. Do you understand how these groups are classified?

- Yes
- No
- Unsure

10. Do these groups influence which CPD activities you will do?

- Yes
- No
- Unsure

11. Not more than 50% of the annual CPD credits required for renewal of registration can be claimed by undertaking Group 1 CPD activities. Should Group 1 activities be limited?

- Yes
- No
- Unsure

12. If you have answered yes to the previous question, please indicate what you believe the limitation should be.

- less than 50%
- more than 50%
- equal to 50%

13. For the following list of CPD activities, please give them a numerical rating between 1 and 5; with 1 indicating MOST preferred and 5 the LEAST preferred.

- Attend a lecture.
- Give a conference presentation.
- Complete an online interactive case study.
- Publish an article in a journal.
- Read a journal article.
- Complete a postgraduate education course.
- View an online lecture.
- Join the board of a local pharmacy committee.
- Read an online journal and complete the MCQ assessment.
- Attend an interactive workshop.
- Introduce a new professional service into your pharmacy.
- View an online interactive lecture.

14. Do you know how to undertake selfdirected learning as part of a structured learning plan?

- Yes
- No
- Unsure

15. Are you using self-directed structured learning plans to guide your CPD activities?

- Always
- Often
- Sometimes
- Never

16. Did you use self-directed structured learning plans before national mandatory CPD was introduced?

- Always
- Often
- Sometimes
- Never

17. Are you recording CPD activities in the correct format required for audit?

- No
- Yes
- Don't know

18. Continuing professional development can also be known as continuing education.

- No
- Yes
- Don't know

The last few questions on this page investigate how you acquire CPD credits.

19. Please show your level of agreement with the following statements. KEY: SA = Strongly Agree, A = Agree, N = Neutral, D = Disagree, SD = Strongly Disagree

- Since CPD became mandatory, I have increased my number of annual CPD activities.

- Since CPD became mandatory, I have participated in a wider variety of CPD activities.
- It will be difficult for me to acquire 40 CPD credits annually.

20. Which of the following make it difficult for you to acquire CPD credits? Tick more than one box if required.

- I have no difficulties in acquiring CPD credits
- Workload
- Unsure what to do.
- Time constraints
- Access to Continuing Education events
- Cost
- Other (please specify)

21. Describe the main difficulty (if any) to obtaining your annual CPD credits.
22. Why is this challenging for you?
23. What has helped you to acquire your annual CPD credits?
24. Are you a member of a professional organisation?

- Yes
- No

25. If you answered 'yes' to the previous question, please state which professional organisation(s) you are a member of.

This now ends the survey on CPD. Thank you for participating.

If you would like to be entered into the prize draw then answer 'Yes' to the next question, otherwise answer 'No' to finish the survey.

26. Would you like to be entered into our prize draw? Two participants will be selected to win a $50 Coles/Myer voucher?

- Yes please
- No thanks

Please enter your e-mail address in the text box and we will contact you if you are selected in the draw.

27. Please note that your e-mail address will be used for the purpose of this draw only and it will be deleted immediately after the winners are selected.

Appendix Survey 2 Questions

Demographics

1. Age:
2. Sex M/F:
3. Single Professional Organisation you most closely identify with … … … … … … … … … …
4. Location (Post code of workplace) (Optional):
5. ITP Provider (Optional): PSA ☐ Guild ☐ NAPE ☐ Other ☐ … … … … … … …
6. University of Study (Optional): …
7. Prior Study/Other Qualifications:
8. Registered Pharmacist: YES/NO (* If NO go to Q 11)
9. Years of Practice: 1–2 ☐ 2–5 ☐ 5–6 ☐ 6–10 ☐ 10–15 ☐ 15+ ☐

10. Currently practising: YES/NO (* If NO go the Q11)
11. Area of Practice Academia ☐ Hospital ☐ Community ☐ Other ☐
12. Hours/week (paid) ... ...

Survey

13. I am familiar with the following documents/resources;

Standards/Framework	Strongly Agree	Agree	Unsure	Disagree	Strongly Disagree
National Competency Standards Framework for Pharmacists in Australia					
Professional Practice Profile for Initial Registration as a Pharmacist					
Australian Qualifications Framework					
Science, Vet, Health Threshold Learning Outcomes					
OLT Pharmacy Threshold Learning Outcomes					

For the remainder of the survey the Competency Standards Framework for Australian Pharmacists will be referred to as the Competency Standards.

14. Do you know what the Competency Standards are? YES/NO/UNSURE
15. Can you describe these in your own words? YES/NO/UNSURE
15a) Description ... ...
16. Have you accessed the Competency Standards document? YES/NO/UNSURE
16a) If YES; Format used; Hard Copy ☐ Online ☐ Both ☐ Unsure ☐
16b) If YES; How often? Nil ☐ Once ☐ Twice ☐ Weekly ☐ Monthly ☐
17. Do you think the Competency Standards are relevant to you now? YES/NO/UNSURE
18. Do you think the Competency Standards will be relevant to you in the future? YES/NO/UNSURE
19. Do you refer to the Competency Standards to compile your CPD? YES/NO/UNSURE
19a) Can you describe any Barriers?
    ... ...
    ... ...
19b) Can you think of any Enablers?
    ... ...
    ... ...

20. Do you refer to the Competency Standards to chart your own progress? YES/NO/UNSURE
20a) If YES; How many times did you refer to the competency standards throughout the year?
    Nil ☐ Once ☐ Twice ☐ Weekly ☐ Monthly ☐
21. How do you use the competency standards currently?

    (a)   Construct CPD Plan
    (b)   Tick the box at registration
    (c)   Reference

22. How do you track your CPD currently?

    (a)   ePortfolio
    (b)   PSA Website

    (c)   Excell doc

    (d)   AuspharmList

    (e)   Other . . . .

23.   In your own experience as a student, do you feel the Competency Standards were introduced to students in the undergraduate or masters programs? YES/NO/UNSURE

23a) Please feel free to add a comment:

24.   In your own experience as an intern, do you feel the Competency Standards informed the intern training program you participated in? YES/NO/UNSURE

24a) Please feel free to add a comment:

25.   Do you think your current students are familiar with the Competency Standards? YES/NO

26.   The following statements refer to various aspects of your practice. I am most interested in obtaining your candid opinions to these statements. Please choose one of five possible responses for each statement about continued competency:

Question	Strongly Agree	Agree	Unsure	Disagree	Strongly Disagree
I can maintain an acceptable standard of practice without attending continuing education programs.					
Continuing education such as self-study or seminars is essential for my work.					
My daily practice is all the continuing education I need.					
I would attend continuing education seminars only if they were required for re-licensure.					
Continuing education is of little importance to my practice.					
My practice would suffer if I did not attend continuing education programs.					

Adapted from [47].

Appendix   Social Media Comments

Pharmacy News (Tessa Hoffman). *Most pharmacists in breach of new CPD rule.* (10 comments) 22 August 2016. Accessed on 23 December 2016 at http://www.pharmacynews.com.au/news/latest-news/most-pharmacists-in-breach-of-new-cpd-rule.

Probably because it is a useless process that has been poorly outlined and explained by the Pharmacy Board. PSA has a CPD planning tool which is laborious and unhelpful. Yet they tell us if we don't use it, we're probably doing it wrong.

Surely we all do CPD that is relevant to our practice, or to practice that we're interested in moving into. Why would we waste our time doing anything else?

We have no time and no motivation for CPD plans, especially since it is all for a pay-packet that we could get at the local supermarket.

For soooo many to not understand means it hasn't been explained very well at all!!!!

The Guild's MYCPD is still developing a tool so that's part of my reasoning of not having a plan as yet .... not going to do the process twice, don't have the time and don't get paid for it .... hard enough to make a buck as it is!!

That's because it is nonsense. I refuse to write a plan and will continue to study and read what takes my fancy or I feel needs refreshing. It's [a] fluid thing—i.e., meet [a] patient with a certain condition and research it.

Pharmacy **2017**, *5*, 12

Attend a conference that takes my fancy. Do a post graduate uni course that presents itself. It's not planned but adjusted to need in an environment of continual learning. Whoever comes up with this crap needs a life and to stop finding more crap for us to do instead of helping patients.

I mean who seriously has the time to sit down and plan their CPD footprint for the next 12 months. Get a life people. I'll take the fine any day. It's not like my $25/hr job is that great anyway. Worse comes to worse I'll just get a job at Bing Lee.

Seems that our regulators have run out of good and worthwhile things to do—and run out of people to annoy all at the same time. Someone or some committee must have needed to justify their ongoing employment. Thus a further load of regulatory bs has been added to that which already exists.

Having worked through the PSA "tool" and having developed a "plan" I am in the compliant 10% and am happy to have given assorted regulators and software "tool" developers something to do for the time being but I wonder what new schemes are being dreamt up to bother us next year and in years to come

That approx. 90% appear not to be compliant tends to demonstrate that the CPD plan and the PGA and PSA tools are bad policy and not acceptable to the majority and that the whole "plan" concept needs to be re-evaluated for real life relevance

Now I assume that the regulators and software developers are actually being paid—unlike the rest of us who must do CPD in our own unpaid time and pay to attend courses etc.—so there's probably little realisation of the financial and social costs of CPD schemes as they apply to the profession as a whole—maybe there needs to be a cost/benefit study into CPD before any more regulatory schemes

When we develop an in-store promotion or a protocol to achieve a desired outcome we plan the event. We start with a need, weed out the non-essential elements and hone the process until we have a desired workable system. The CPD plan is nothing but an extension of that process. It is to ensure we develop in the best path possible so that we can deliver our knowledge, remain focused and enthused in our profession and not wander off on unproductive tangents. The only difficulty at the moment is the means to develop this, just as professional bodies are also still formulating, but we should be able to jots down personal guideline and ideas as we wait patiently for a definitive checklist or table. Good luck with yours. I realise how challenging it is as I believe that even though I have one, I need to continually monitor and work on it as situations and demands on my talents change.

I think a bigger concern is the current expectation for plan + CPD exceeds all other areas of allied health ... whilst getting paid less.

Anyone who has any clinical responsibility where there recommendation are held to account by medical teams does this automatically. It is not challenging it is a waste of time.

Actually I need sit down and partake in dribble. I learn, and study and do plenty of CPD but I don't waste time writing a plan. I don't feel lacking in any areas to plan. Things present themselves and it is only then you realise you don't know enough so you research it. If you see an interesting conference you do it, as CPD pops up on various websites you follow what takes your fancy. A course comes up that is relevant you do it, I don't waste time planning and documenting and fluffing about, I get on with it. I don't waste time recording interventions either as we do to many being in a medical centre and time is precious.

Over documentation and fakery are the nonsense bull dust of the modern world. Wasting time, money and intentions.

Some people might operate that way and it works for them but for me I feel like screaming every time a new rule is introduced to complicate life.

No time for this kind of craps. I have my own plan in my head. I don't need to write it down as proof to show the board. Pharmacists are not kids and the Board is not our parents. I don't waste my time that I can use to treat my patients. At home, I need time for my family. Otherwise, my wife would divorce me. Believe it or not, it is true. Will the Board pay me the divorce fee? If not, then leave all pharmacists alone. With only $25 an hour, don't ask too much from pharmacists. Otherwise, everyone will quit and work for Aldi or BingLee. Same money, but less responsibilities and less crap.

Pharmacy **2017**, *5*, 12

Pharmacy News (Tessa Hoffman) *Six things to know about your CPD plan.* (22 Comments) 23/08/2016. Accessed on 23/12/2016 at http://www.pharmacynews.com.au/news/latest-news/six-things-to-know-about-your-cpd-plan.

When did Intern supervising get taken off? If that's the case, I have a lot of hours to do in the next month.

The template is headed 'Plan/Record'. Are we required to make a record of the past year or a plan for the next year?

Seriously, could there be any more work they want to load on us for the measly $27/hr???!!! I can get that wage at Aldi without all this headache.

Pharmacy is a dead end job!!! Get out while you can.

I really find this ridiculous—I refuse to write a plan. Do they not realise people will write what ever and just dribble in then go about what they do normally anyway? Just like QCPP? All words and fluff and no substance.

I do so much CPD more than I do work actually and spend considerable money on it. I refuse to write a plan. It's ridiculous. I can now either lie like most people will or send a copy of my new postgraduate degree and say this should bloody cover it. It makes my blood boil. I think everyone should refuse. They can't deregister us all

Absolutely agree. I doubt that anyone who actually works full time in the profession was involved in the development of this rubbish.

No, I don't think I'll be doing this. Undertake and record my mandated yearly points, that's what I'll do.

How do you decide what CPD to do? Is it anything that is timely and convenient, or to fill gaps in your knowledge and skills?

Thanks to HMR caps, expensive CPD events/post grad courses were the first thing I culled despite their clinical relevance and profession expansion. Clinical knowledge and practice is not monetarily rewarded, nor is it recognised by the PGA, AACP, PSA in terms of career expansion .... so why put any time and money into it?

Knowledge is power. And that can bring rewards. Think for example about the pilot sites for health care homes announced yesterday. How will practices choose a pharmacist to be part of the HC home? It will be based on your reputation and capacity to contribute to the team. They will be looking for pharmacists with a high level of clinical knowledge.

No, it will be decided as all these things are by informal networks between Pharmacy owners and GP practices. Employee Clinical Pharmacist input = Zero

Knowledge is power, at least in most industries. Absolutely reputation will help you gain a position such as this. However, I'm not holding my breath regarding the HC homes until I see the remuneration offered. Only then can we gauge how the government values clinical pharmacist input. With HMRs being one of the most valuable services available...culling them to me sends a pretty clear message. This move was met with very little resistance from all pharmacy bodies (including accreditation bodies) which sends an even bigger message. This would not have happened in any other industry. So it would appear clinical knowledge gives you very little power where it matters most.

On a side note anyone know the role of the AACP? They didn't release a position statement when the caps were announced. Their fees haven't decreased since the caps. All I can see is that they release an occasional newsletter and email regarding upcoming expensive CPD programs they are holding to receive more money (I'm yet to see a medical consultant on the list of speakers, who often offer far greater insight into medication use in their field than a pharmacist).

The only thing Pharmacy owners ever ask prospective Pharmacist employees is how many scripts can you dispense per hour. No one cares about your clinical skills or knowledge nor is it reflected in the Pharmacy award which has become not only the legal minimum but the de facto pay rate for many.

I never, ever, ever do the business-related CPD. It has SFA to do with my practice as a pharmacist and to be frank is insulting that it is scored the same in terms of development in learning about a new drug class, treatment regimen, or health topic.

If I come across a topic I feel I don't know enough about—that's my CPD. Hard to plan and map that, because like Uncle Don said "There's things you know you don't know, and there's things you don't know you don't know".

That is what people will do regardless—they will just pretend to plan it at the end of the year. I also feel you don't know what you want to learn until you realise you don't know it—then you immediately rectify the situation. Such as coming across a drug or a condition you need to know about but don't. You don't plan to study it later in the year to open google and get to it. You target your CPD to your interests and practice anyway.

I understand some people might like to operate that way but for me, useless meaningless paperwork I will not partake of.

Those that are not keeping will not change their practice either—They will just lie.

I do CPD based on (admittedly, self-ID'd) knowledge gaps. Personal and family commitments mean that for me a plan is too constricting (ie. do x at time y), and sometimes things that I thought I needed to study two months ago don't actually require the active study I thought they did because of the passive intake of information (like Zika for instance—bits and pieces over months complete the picture, rather than a block of time to swot the subject). I'm taking a calculated risk and if I'm audited that's fine, that's the game.

Pharmacy News (Tessa Hoffman) *Pharmacists Lash Out* (16 Comments), 24/8/2016. Accessed on 23 December 2016 at; http://www.pharmacynews.com.au/news/latest-news/pharmacists-lash-out-against-new-cpd-rule.

All it will do is make people consider what the most relevant training is for them .... and then make them reconcile that against competency standards. And then make them document what they did. And then make them document how it changed their practice. No, that won't be time consuming at all ....

Why can't pharmacy just go back to voluntary CPD? Instead of this "Big Brother with the Big (deregistration) Stick" approach.

Umm, I just made my plan; "Get to 40 CPD points" Isn't that sufficient?

I think this the ultimate "nanny" phenomena. If we accrue 40 points, subject finished requirements met. If you can't meet the 40 points without a plan you shouldn't be a registered pharmacist "GO HARD OR GO HOME".

Anyone with any level of clinical accountability who is not actively seeking to fill knowledge gaps and expand should not be practicing. Direct HMR referrals uncapped would assist with this over "CPD plans" ... call itself auditing by GPs. Written plans are useless. Most will be completed in hindsight based on what was completed earlier in the year.

As pharmacy continues to get raped this plan is ridiculous! CPD is expensive and time consuming as it is. Accredited pharmacists need to complete 60 CPD points .... can only see 20 patients a month and now require a plan! What a joke!!!!

Here's perspective physio CPD is 20 hours a year

Since we are scientists and deal with evidence-based therapies, can AHPRA or the Pharmacy Board provide us with studies that prove that pharmacists with a CPD plan perform better or are more up to date than those who don't have a CPD plan?

Time and time again we see examples of how some moron trying to justify their salary and position on the board come up with some stupid idea that gets supported by other idiots who think they are actually more important than they really are. The new requirement for a compulsory CPD plan is yet another example.

I've yet to meet one pharmacist who believes in the idea who doesn't have some other agenda they're working on (e.g., seeking a position on the board or some academic position because they themselves can't stand working in community pharmacy anymore).

All the negative comments from other readers to date will as usual be ignored. The point that our pay is a joke is always rebutted with the argument that we should be happy to be working at all or that we are lucky to be in a respected job. Well I've got news for you—pharmacy is definitely not what it used to be. The only people I feel worse for are the pharmacy assistants who work their backsides off for the lowest pay rates in the country.

We are all expected to perform a lot more for a lot less these days and sell out our dignity in the process (e.g., Generic substation/"value plus", discount pharmacy models, etc.). This is apparently the better working standard that is the trade-off for the low pay we're expected to be content with.

Back to the compulsory CPD plan debate—it won't achieve anything other than waste pharmacists' time. The idiot who drafted it will somehow put a spin on it with fancy stats to indicate how it will improve pharmacy practice but it will be a lie. Every pharmacist I've spoken to has indicated that if push comes to shove and they have to do it the only way they can draw up a plan is in retrospect i.e., do the compulsory CPD during the year to get the points then work backwards to come up with a plan. How else could it work if you don't even know what CPD activities are available at the start of the year? So if most pharmacists are planning to come up with the plan in this way how does it achieve anything other than waste all our valuable time. And while on the topic of time could someone please work out what our actual hourly rates are after factoring in all the hours we spend on compulsory CPD as well as the money spent to attend activities, pay for annual registration, professional indemnity insurance, and so on and so on.

Pharmacy is the joke among all university studied professions!

Year after year I see disillusioned young men and women come out into the pharmacy workforce regretting their choice of career.

For myself I only work in pharmacy on weekends because the penalty rates (while they still exist) at least make it bearable. I have a second job in another industry during the week so that I can maintain a half decent lifestyle otherwise I would fall below the poverty line like all our poor pharmacy assistants.

I'm a casual locum .... I'm stuffed if I can satisfy the Boards multi-level requirements in their "PLAN" .... I have had no problem obtaining 100 plus Points annually since CPD started, you can't tell me I'm not trying!!

CPD's should only be used as a punishment system for pharmacists who have demonstrated negligent practices. Everyone else has demonstrated that the knowledge they acquired studying to become b a pharmacist or due to their experience as being a pharmacist is sufficient enough for the health care needs of their workplace and demographic.

I do believe we need to keep up-to-date and do a lot of CPD to [keep] up to speed and because I like to learn but these plans are just bull shittery concocted up by some numpty with ocd.

The board is dreaming if they think their $26 pharmacists will spend a single minute on this rubbish. Hell being deregistered could be a blessing in disguise. You'll probably earn more elsewhere anyways.

No time for this kind of crap. I have my own plan in my head. I don't need to write it down as proof to show the board. Pharmacists are not kids and the Board is not our parents. I don't waste my time that I can use to treat my patients. At home, I need time for my family. Otherwise, my wife would divorce me. Will the Board pay me the divorce fee? If not, then leave all pharmacists alone. With only $25 an hour, don't ask too much from pharmacists. Otherwise, everyone will quit and work for Aldi or BingLee. Same money, but less responsibilities and less craps.

If the board has time to audit pharmacists regarding the CPD plan, I am wondering why they don't audit Chemist Warehouse for compliance of Pharmacy Standards? Pharmacists in Chemist Warehouse don't counsel patients at all. It is not their fault, but the fault of the founders of Chemist Warehouse.

Pharmacists with no CPD plan do not cause any harm to patients, but Chemist Warehouse giving out medications without counseling would cause harm.

I myself don't have time to write down the CPD plan. I won't do it until the Board provide proof that all other pharmacists have the plan. I have the same plan as "Ain't nobody got time for dat" in this forum, namely: Get to 40 CPD points. Simple!!!

AJP.com.au (Sheshtyn Paola) *Pharmacy Board responds to CPD plan uproar* (7 Comments), 29/08/2016. Accessed on 23/12/2016 at https://ajp.com.au/news/pharmacy-board-responds-cpd-plan-uproar/.

Can I point out that a plan is personal to you and your circumstances. It can be simple or complicated and you sure don't need a workshop to make one. I'm pretty sure you are not going to be marked on it! Bit of common sense needed in this discussion.

Exactly, it's mindless busy work.

The revised registration standards and CPD guidelines followed a rigorous public consultation process

I agree that we were informed early enough of the need to have a CPD plan, however I strongly dispute the suggestion that this followed a "rigorous consultation process". Who exactly was consulted. I certainly wasn't, nor was I aware that there was a consultation process.

Bureaucratic time wasting. Next they'll have us write a protocol for attending CPD events, requiring a plan on where we sit, when we started sitting and how it impacted our learning by sitting in that spot.

SHPA also has a package of material to support members prepare a learning plan—including an online presentation that explains in detail how to develop a learning plan and competency grids for a range of pharmacist roles.

References

1. Nash, R.; Chalmers, L.; Brown, N.; Jackson, S.; Peterson, G. An international review of program wide use of competency standards in pharmacy education. *Pharm. Educ. J.* **2015**, *15*, 131–141.
2. National Competency Standards Framework for Pharmacists in Australia. 2010. Available online: http://www.psa.org.au/supporting-practice/national-competency-standards (accessed on 30 January 2015).
3. Pharmaceutical Society of Australia. Professional Practice Standards. 2010. Available online: https://www.psa.org.au/supporting-practice/professional-practice-standards (accessed on 12 June 2016).
4. Australian Commission on Safety and Quality in Health Care. National Safety and Quality Health Service Standards. 2012. Available online: https://www.safetyandquality.gov.au/our-work/accreditation-and-the-nsqhs-standards/resources-to-implement-the-nsqhs-standards/#NSQHS-Standards (accessed on 22 February 2017).
5. Ryan, J. Continuous professional development along the continuum of lifelong learning. *Nurse Educ. Today* **2003**, *23*, 498–508. [CrossRef]
6. Rouse, M.J. Continuing professional development in pharmacy. *Am. J. Health Syst. Pharm.* **2004**, *61*, 2069–2076. [PubMed]
7. Driesen, A.; Verbeke, K.; Simoens, S.; Laekeman, G. International Trends in Lifelong Learning for Pharmacists. *Am. J. Pharm. Educ.* **2007**, *71*, 52. [CrossRef] [PubMed]
8. Meštrović, A.; Rouse, M.J. Pillars and Foundations of Quality for Continuing Education in Pharmacy. *Am. J. Pharm. Educ.* **2015**, *79*, 45. [CrossRef] [PubMed]
9. Konstantinides, G. Continuing Professional Development: The role of a regulatory board in promoting lifelong learning. *Innov. Pharm.* **2010**, *1*, 14.
10. Institute of Medicine. Redesigning Continuing Education in the Healthcare Professions. 2009. Available online: http://www.policymed.com/2009/12/institute-of-medicine-redesigning-continuing-education-in-the-health-professions.html (accessed on 13 January 2017).
11. Siemens, G. Connectivism: A Learning Theory for the Digital Age. Available online: http://er.dut.ac.za/bitstream/handle/123456789/69/Siemens_2005_Connectivism_A_learning_theory_for_the_digital_age.pdf?sequence=1&isAllowed=y (accessed on 22 February 2017).

12. Wiedenmayer, K.; Summers, R.S.; Mackie, C.A.; Gous, A.G.; Everard, M.; Tromp, D. *Developing Pharmacy Practice: A Focus on Patient Care: Handbook*; World Health Organization and International Pharmaceutical Federation: Hague, The Netherlands, 2006; p. 15.

13. Pharmacy Board of Australia. Guidelines on Continuing Professional Development. 2015. Available online: http://www.pharmacyboard.gov.au/News/2015-10-30-registration-standards.aspx (accessed on 21 December 2015).

14. Kolb, D.A. *Experiential Learning: Experience as the Source of Learning and Development*; Kolb, D.A., Ed.; Prentice Hall: Englewood Cliffs, NJ, USA, 1984.

15. Pharmacy Board of Australia. Continuing Professional Development (CPD) FAQ. Available online: http://www.pharmacyboard.gov.au/Codes-Guidelines/FAQ/CPD-FAQ.aspx (accessed on 9 December 2016).

16. Biggs, J.; Tang, C. *Teaching for Quality Learning at University: What the Student Does*, 4th ed.; McGraw-Hill Education: Berkshire, UK, 2011.

17. Harden, R.; Crosby, J.; Davis, M. AMEE guide No. 14: Outcome-based education: Part 1—An introduction to outcome education. *Med. Teach.* **1999**, *21*, 7–14.

18. Australian Government Department of Education and Training. *Higher Education Standards Framework (Threshold Standards)*; Australian Government Department of Education and Training: Canberra, Australia, 2015; pp. 4 and pp. 7–8.

19. Australian Pharmacy Council. Accreditation Standards for Pharmacy Programs in Australia and New Zealand. Available online: http://pharmacycouncil.org.au/content/index.php?id=17 (accessed on 26 February 2015).

20. Jackson, D. *The Contribution of Work-Integrated Learning to Undergraduate Employability Skill Outcomes*; New Zealand Association for Cooperative Education: Hamilton, New Zealand, 2013; pp. 99–115.

21. Freudenberg, B.; Brimble, M.; Cameron, C.; MacDonald, K.L.; English, D.M. I am what I am: Am I? The development of self-efficacy through work integrated learning. *Int. J. Pedagog. Curric. (Sect. Int. J. Learn.)* **2013**, *19*, 177–192.

22. Wilkens, S.; Tucci, J. Group Project—Learning Research and Generic Skills for Life beyond University. *Pharmacy* **2014**, *2*, 65. [CrossRef]

23. Kehoe, A.; Goudzwaard, M. ePortfolios, Badges, and the Whole Digital Self: How Evidence-Based Learning Pedagogies and Technologies Can Support Integrative Learning and Identity Development. *Theory Pract.* **2015**, *54*, 343–351. [CrossRef]

24. Chen, H.; Grocott, L.; Kehoe, A. Changing Records of Learning Through Innovations in Pedagogy and Technology. Educause Review. 2016. Available online: http://er.educause.edu/articles/2016/3/changing-records-of-learning-through-innovations-in-pedagogy-and-technology (accessed on 31 March 2016).

25. Oliver, B.; von Konsky, B.R.; Jones, S.; Ferns, S.; Tucker, B. Curtin's iPortfolio: Facilitating student achievement of graduate attributes within and beyond the formal curriculum. *Learn. Communities Int. J. Learn. Soc. Contexts* **2009**, *2*, 4–15.

26. Scott, G. *Powerful Assessment in Higher Education: Identification of Case Studies of Productive Approaches within and Beyond Australia*; Australian Office of Learning and Teaching: Sydney, Australia, 2015; p. 4.

27. Fernandez, N.; Dory, V.; Ste-Marie, L.G.; Chaput, M.; Charlin, B.; Boucher, A. Varying conceptions of competence: An analysis of how health sciences educators define competence. *Med. Educ.* **2012**, *46*, 357–365. [CrossRef] [PubMed]

28. Creswell, J. *Research Design Qualitative, Quantitative and Mixed Methods Approaches*, 2nd ed.; SAGE Publications, Inc.: Thousand Oaks, CA, USA, 2013.

29. Denscombe, M. *The Good Research Guide; Surveys and Sampling*; Open University Press: Maidenhead, UK, 2010.

30. Liamputtong, P. *Research Methods in Health: Foundations for Evidence-Based Practice*, 2nd ed.; Oxford University Press: Melbourne, Australia, 2013.

31. Nash, R.E.; Chalmers, L.; Stupans, I.; Brown, N. Knowledge, use and perceived relevance of a profession's Competency Standards; implications for Pharmacy Education. *Int. J. Pharm. Pract.* **2016**, *24*, 390–402. [CrossRef] [PubMed]

32. Braun, V.; Clarke, V. Using thematic analysis in psychology. *Qual. Res. Psychol.* **2006**, *3*, 77–101. [CrossRef]

33. Australian Health Practitioner Regulation Agency. The Australian Health Practitioner Regulation Agency and the National Boards, Reporting on the National Registration and Accreditation Scheme: Annual Report 2010–2011. Available online: http://www.ahpra.gov.au/Publications/Corporate-publications/Annual-reports.aspx (accessed on 22 December 2016).

34. Thompson, W.; Nissen, L.; Hayward, K. Australian pharmacists' understanding of their continuing professional development obligations. *Aust. J. Pharm.* **2013**, *94*, 58–60. [CrossRef]

35. Australian Qualifications Framework Council. *Australian Qualifications Framework Second Edition I*; Department of Industry, Science, Research and Tertiary Education: Adelaide, Australia, 2013.

36. Hattie, J. *Visible Learning: A Synthesis of Over 800 Meta-Analyses Relating to Achievement*; Taylor and Francis: Hoboken, NJ, USA, 2008.

37. Nash, R.; Stupans, I.; Chalmers, L.; Brown, N. Traffic Light Report provides a new technique for Assurance of Learning. *J. Learn. Des.* **2016**, *9*, 37–54. [CrossRef]

38. Donyai, P.; Herbert, R.Z.; Denicolo, P.M.; Alexander, A.M. British pharmacy professionals' beliefs and participation in continuing professional development: A review of the literature. *Int. J. Pharm. Pract.* **2011**, *19*, 290–317. [CrossRef] [PubMed]

39. Collins, J. Lifelong Learning in the 21st Century and Beyond. *RadioGraphics* **2009**, *29*, 613–622. [CrossRef] [PubMed]

40. Bembenutty, H. Introduction: Self-regulation of learning in postsecondary education. *New Direct. Teach. Learn.* **2011**, *2011*, 3–8. [CrossRef]

41. Boud, D.; Falchikov, N. Aligning assessment with long-term learning. *Assess. Eval. High. Educ.* **2006**, *31*, 399–413. [CrossRef]

42. Dopp, A.L.; Moulton, J.R.; Rouse, M.J.; Trewet, C.B. A five-state continuing professional development pilot program for practicing pharmacists. *Am. J. Pharm. Educ.* **2010**, *74*, 28. [CrossRef] [PubMed]

43. Hughes, C.; Barrie, S. Influences on the assessment of graduate attributes in higher education. *Assess. Eval. High. Educ.* **2010**, *35*, 325–334.

44. Austin, Z.; Gregory, P. Evaluating the Accuracy of Pharmacy Students' Self-Assessment Skills. *Am. J. Pharm. Educ.* **2007**, *71*, 1–89. [CrossRef]

45. Laaksonen, R.; Bates, I.; Duggan, C. Training, clinical medication review performance and self-assessed competence: Investigating influences. *Pharm. Educ.* **2007**, *7*, 257–265. [CrossRef]

46. Pfleger, D.; McHattie, L.; Diack, H.; McCaig, D.; Stewart, D. Views, attitudes and self-assessed training needs of Scottish community pharmacists to public health practice and competence. *Pharm. World Sci.* **2008**, *30*, 801–809. [CrossRef] [PubMed]

47. Schack, D.; Hepler, C. Modification of Hall's Professionalism Scale for Use with Pharmacists. *Am. J. Pharm. Educ.* **1979**, *43*, 98–104.

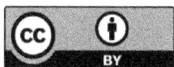

pharmacy

MDPI

Article

Competence-Based Curricula in the Context of Bologna and EU Higher Education Policy

Howard Davies

European University Association, Avenue de l'Yser 24 Ijserlaan, Brussels B-1040, Belgium;
howard.davies@eua.be; Tel.: +44-7780-700-648

Academic Editor: Jeffrey Atkinson
Received: 16 January 2017; Accepted: 23 March 2017; Published: 26 March 2017

Abstract: At the turn of the century European higher education policy became twin-track. The Bologna Process was launched and ran alongside developments in European legislation. Both tracks displayed a preoccupation with competences, in relation both to citizenship and to labour market needs. Scrutiny of important policy texts (Key Competences, the European Qualifications Framework, ECTS, the Bologna three-cycle degree structure) shows that 'competence' has never been given a precise and secure definition. Only very recently has the term entered the discourse of EU legislation on the recognition of professional qualifications. Current work on competence-based curricula in sectoral professions, including pharmacy, has helped bring the two policy tracks into closer alignment. The examples of competences identified in specific professional contexts can assist EU and Bologna policy-makers as they confront future challenges.

Keywords: competence; profession; curriculum; policy

1. Introduction

European higher education policy follows two tracks. The first, in historical terms, is the vision elaborated over many years by the European Commission. A host of Communications and working documents have been produced, which may or may not have been subsequently enshrined in legislation. This would have depended on their acceptability to the legislative bodies—Council and Parliament—but also on the degree of legal competence enjoyed by the European Community or the European Union at any given moment in time.

Since the Treaty of Maastricht in 1992, education has become much more strictly the province of Member States (MSs); the capacity of action of the EU institutions is now that of a 'complementary competence', undertaking at EU level that which cannot be achieved by MSs acting independently.

The second track is the Bologna Process, an inter-governmental action programme dating from the Sorbonne Declaration of 1998 and the Bologna Declaration of 1999. By 2010, the Process had put in place the European Higher Education Area (EHEA). The EHEA is effectively co-regulated by the 48 signatory countries (or regions of countries) together with European-level bodies representing social partners and sectoral stakeholders (institutions, students, quality assurance agencies). It has a legal base, the Lisbon Recognition Convention (LRC), although in practice the relevant legislation is enacted by the signatory countries within their own territories.

The two tracks are not independent of each other. The European Commission participates in summit meetings and is also a member of the Bologna Follow-Up Group (BFUG) which manages Bologna Process business between the bi- or triennial meetings of the 48 ministers. It has funded a number of the Bologna Process initiatives.

But neither are the two tracks fully integrated or geo-politically congruent. The Bologna Process covers countries from Iceland to Russia, from Norway to Armenia. EU legislation extends to the 28 MSs and the three countries in the European Economic Area—Iceland, Liechtenstein and Norway. Their relationship, however, has evolved through time, to the extent that it is now possible to speak of a gradual convergence, at least as far as the recognition of professional qualifications and the development of competence-based curricula are concerned.

For over the past ten years, a number of professions have embarked on competence-based curricula as a way of consolidating both professional expertise and public trust. In many instances—medical doctors, dentists, nurses, pharmacists and architects—the emphasis has been on refocusing the basic training prescribed by EU legislation on the recognition of professional qualifications [1]. In doing so, the professions—and notably the academics in the professions—have worked within the parameters of the Bologna Process. Their work has been located at the point of convergence of two related trends: the shift from teacher-centred training to student-centred learning, orchestrated by the Bologna Process; and the determination to integrate the EU labour market following the financial crisis of 2008.

2. Europe Pre-Bologna

EU employment policy did not emerge fully-formed in the aftermath of 2008. Article 57.1 of the Treaty of Rome (1957) laid the foundation stone for current legislation on the recognition of professional qualifications, based on the free movement of citizens and the drive to create a Single Market. While it led to the raft of Directives on seven sectoral professions (including that of the pharmacist) in the late 1970s, it did not represent the birth of a higher education policy. That particular initiative had already been taken, relatively independently, in the early part of the same decade. Anne Corbett offers a detailed and insightful account of what she refers to as the 'creation of a policy domain' [2] by the 'policy entrepreneurs' who created the ERASMUS programme of student and staff mobility and the COMETT support for university-enterprise partnerships.

In general, however, European higher educational policy statements [3] in the late 1980s and early 1990s mainly concern mobility, quality assessment, and distance learning. Labour market considerations are reserved for the vocational education and training (VET) sector. The Treaty of Maastricht in 1992 checked the flow of educational initiatives by confining the European institutions to a complementary role, the principal responsibility for higher education resting with MSs. This made it more challenging to implement the conclusions of the Study Group on Education and Training set up by Commissioner Cresson in 1995, which stressed the importance of adopting a 'strategy of continually raising competence levels' [4].

It was the perceived need to re-assert a transnational policy frame that prompted France, supported by Germany, Italy and the UK, to resort to inter-governmental action in 1998. This was the Sorbonne Declaration, which one year later mutated into the Bologna Process. It proposed concerted structural change, the facilitation of mobility by credit accumulation and transfer, and a framework of lifelong learning. It was then that the flow of policy-making divided into the two tracks described above. Between them, the ability to cross-refer was not strong. The Bologna Process involved ministers of education in a series of commitments, which those from European Community MSs were able to echo in meetings of the Education Council. However, coming from governments organised in different ways and according to different priorities, they enjoyed varying degrees of collaboration, at European level, with their peers who sat in the Competitiveness Council and who were responsible for research, national economies and labour markets. It was left to the Commission to take up the challenge put down by Edith Cresson's Study Group and to address the question of competences.

3. Key Competences in the European Union

The ambitious Lisbon Strategy, with its oft-quoted aim—"to become the most dynamic and competitive knowledge-based economy in the world by 2010 capable of sustainable economic growth with more and better jobs and greater social cohesion and respect for the environment"—languished at first. The Wim Kok report of 2004 [5] subsequently left no room for doubting that the strategy had run into difficulty. The European Commission responded with a Communication on *Mobilising the brainpower of Europe: enabling universities to make their full contribution to the Lisbon strategy* [6] in 2005.

Yet already in 2003, in their joint interim report on *Education and Training 2010: the success of the Lisbon Strategy hinges on urgent reforms* [7], the Commission and the Council had bemoaned the fact that 'nearly 20% of young people fail to acquire key **competences** [8]':

> Everyone needs to acquire a minimum set of **competences** in order to learn, work and achieve fulfilment in a knowledge-driven society and economy. They include traditional key **competences** (reading, writing and numbers) and the newer ones (comprising foreign languages, entrepreneurship, interpersonal and civic **competences**, and **competences** in the new information and communication technologies). However, in the fundamental domain of reading, 17.2% of young Europeans aged under 15 do not have the minimum **competence** required […]

This was to become a familiar refrain. In 2006, the Commission duly published a list of *Key Competences* which was then adopted as a formal Recommendation [9]. Ten in number, the competences were the following:

- communication in the mother tongue;
- communication in foreign languages;
- competences in maths, science and technology;
- digital competence;
- learning to learn;
- interpersonal, intercultural and social competences, and civic competence;
- entrepreneurship;
- cultural expression.

They were to be attained by all citizens by the end of their initial education and training. Without them, the scope for personal fulfilment and social cohesion would be curtailed. It was nevertheless labour market considerations that drove the Commission's initiative.

The Lisbon Agenda of 2000 had been predicated on the principle that competitiveness and cohesion were not mutually exclusive, as well as on the presumption that the EU would thrive by generating knowledge which could be monetised by its transformation into manufactured goods in low-wage economies, notably China. If Europe were to sustain itself as a high-skill, high-wage society, its citizens would have to be educated and trained to the appropriate level—on a lifelong basis. Hence the generic character given to the competences: they were multifunctional and transferable.

The competences were not, however, entirely free-floating. If left to the political will of MSs acting in their own pressurised policy environments, the prospect of uniform application would be at risk. It was necessary to tie the competences into the overarching framework of the European Qualifications Framework for lifelong learning [10] (EQF).

This was done primarily by ensuring that both Recommendations—Key Competences and EQF—were based on compatible definitions of competence. This was a significant step. For native speakers of English, the notion of competence features in common parlance; speakers are nevertheless aware that it implies value judgements which can vary widely.

A workable definition in Euro-English would have to be sufficiently supple to accommodate the intuitions of *compétence*, *Kompetenz*, and so on. The solution adopted was to give it the status of an umbrella concept, under which a bundle of attributes could be gathered:

- In the context of the Key Competences, a **competence** is a 'combination of knowledge, skills and attitudes appropriate to the context' [9] (Annex to Recommendation 2006/962/EC).
- In the EQF, '**competence** means the proven ability to use knowledge, skills and personal, social and/or methodological abilities, in work or study situations and in professional and personal

development. In the context of the European Qualifications Framework, **competence** is described in terms of responsibility and autonomy' [10] (Annex to Recommendation on EQF).

4. Competences in EU Legislation on the Recognition of Professional Qualifications

How do these developments translate into the Directives which apply to the sectoral professions? Only indirectly, it must be said, if at all. With respect to pharmacy [11], the term 'competence' appears nowhere.

Article 45.2 of Directive 2005/36/EC lists seven 'activities':

(a) preparation of the pharmaceutical form of medicinal products;
(b) manufacture and testing of medicinal products;
(c) testing of medicinal products in a laboratory for the testing of medicinal products;
(d) storage, preservation and distribution of medicinal products at the wholesale stage;
(e) preparation, testing, storage and supply of medicinal products in pharmacies open to the public;
(f) preparation, testing, storage and dispensing of medicinal products in hospitals;
(g) provision of information and advice on medicinal products.

The amended Directive 2013/55/EU subsequently re-phrased (e) to read: 'supply, preparation, testing, storage, distribution and dispensing of safe and efficacious medicinal products of the required quality in pharmacies open to the public'. It amplified (f) to read: 'preparation, testing, storage and dispensing of safe and efficacious medicinal products of the required quality in hospitals'. It also amplified (g) to read: 'provision of information and advice on medicinal products as such, including on their appropriate use'. Finally, it added three further 'activities':

(h) reporting of adverse reactions of pharmaceutical products to the competent authorities;
(i) personalised support for patients who administer their medication;
(j) contribution to local or national public health campaigns.

'Activity', however, is a term which appears in neither of the two definitions of competence cited earlier. Moreover, it is clear that only effective safeguards will prevent incompetent persons from engaging in the activities listed. To this end, the Directive prescribes appropriate supplementary professional experience. Article 44.3 renders the practice of the activities conditional upon 'the following knowledge and skills':

(a) adequate knowledge of medicines and the substances used in the manufacture of medicines;
(b) adequate knowledge of pharmaceutical technology and the physical, chemical, biological and microbiological testing of medicinal products;
(c) adequate knowledge of the metabolism and the effects of medicinal products and of the action of toxic substances, and of the use of medicinal products;
(d) adequate knowledge to evaluate scientific data concerning medicines in order to be able to supply appropriate information on the basis of this knowledge;
(e) adequate knowledge of the legal and other requirements associated with the pursuit of pharmacy.

With the exception of the few amendments made in 2013, the specified 'activities', as well as the 'knowledge and skills', follow the wording of Article 1 and 2 of Directive 85/432/EEC [12], wording which in 2005 was twenty years old. Only minimal scrutiny is required to ascertain that the five bodies of knowledge make reference to one single elliptically expressed ability and to no 'skills' whatever.

The wording now goes back thirty-two years—but the preoccupation with competence-based curricula is comparatively recent. How is it that academic and professional bodies in sectoral professions have only latterly begun to concern themselves with competence, when they have long been exercised over the relationship of theory to practice?

Partly the answer lies in their anxiety about patient safety, which has grown as a result of demographic trends and the expansion of patient and professional mobility across EU internal borders. Partly it is due to the influence of the Bologna Process.

Thanks to its mobility instruments—notably the Diploma Supplement—Bologna brought a transparency to curricula which had not existed before. Professional mobility, although underwritten by Directives, had previously operated on the basis of trust. While this trust was not wholly blind, it appeared not to prompt scrutiny of the content of 'foreign' curricula. But as the EU enlarged from 2004 onwards, and as the volume of cross-border professional and patient mobility increased, healthcare stakeholders grew more sensitive to the need for the effective quality assurance of training programmes—their curriculum development, their delivery, and their accreditation.

Problems then became apparent and, with them, a certain resistance to recognition. A report commissioned by the European Parliament in 2009 repeatedly stressed MSs' lack of trust in each other's education systems. It pithily concluded that 'if the MSs could trust each other's education systems and believe that a child nurse is well educated in the EU, regardless of the formal degree he or she has obtained, there might be fewer problems with recognition of professional qualifications' [13] (p. 65).

The lack of trust helped prompt the Commission make provision in the amended Directive for 'common training frameworks' (CTF). Article 49a.1 allows training programmes designed by one third of Member States (i.e., currently ten) to be subject to automatic recognition, if based on a 'common set of minimum knowledge, skills and **competences** necessary for the pursuit of a specific profession' or of a specialty related to one of the sectoral professions. Hospital pharmacists fall into the latter category. Led by the European Association of Hospital Pharmacists (EAHP), they currently lead the field in the development of a CTF and are mapping the competences required in the advanced practice of hospital pharmacy in Europe [14].

Two factors are of note here. First, the amended Directive requires all CTFs to be based on the levels of the EQF, in order to ensure readability across the countries that have referenced their national qualifications frameworks to it.

Secondly, the concept of competence now sits alongside knowledge and skills as an apparently separate category. Notwithstanding the scrubbing to which all EU legal texts are subject, 'competence' has lost its umbrella function as well as, accordingly, its utility as a term with an established legal usage.

Loss of textual cohesion is not quite the same as incoherence, since some sense clearly survives. The looseness of expression is nonetheless worrying, particularly in view of recent developments which show the European Commission to be adopting an ever more 'technicist' approach to education and training in its promotion of employability.

5. The Potential for Competence-Based Curricula in Pharmacy

Despite the introduction of CTFs, it remains true that the 'core' pharmacy Articles of the Directive do not explicitly encourage the development of competence-based curricula. But to what extent do they inhibit it? Recital 25 alludes to the 'coordinated minimum range of activities' to be covered in pharmacy training, clearly indicating that MSs may go beyond the minimum. They may, therefore, choose to require additional activities, which they may frame in terms of competences if they so choose.

Furthermore, the Directive, while prescribing a minimum of five years full-time training, does not lay down a precise number of hours. Nor does it, in Annex 5.6.2, give a precise quantification of the required 'balance' between theoretical and practical work. Moreover, it allows the five years to be expressed in ECTS credits, which embrace contact hours, projects, practical work, placements and private study.

On the face of it, it would appear—at least to the non-pharmacist author of this article—that EU legislation puts no impediment in the way of competence-based curriculum designers. They may proceed with as much freedom as their national regulatory framework allows. To secure a firmer transnational structure for collaboration, they have three recourses: first, the CTFs already mentioned:

secondly, the review of the Directive in 2019; thirdly, applying pressure to the Bologna Process to build stronger consensus around the concept of competence.

6. Competences in the Bologna Process

To what extent is the unstable definition of competence mirrored in its occurrences in the Bologna Declaration of 1999 and in the eight ministerial communiqués which have followed it [15]? They reveal an initial focus on competences associated with citizenship. This focus never entirely disappears, but weakens as the emphasis on lifelong labour market relevance grows. At the most recent ministerial conference—in Yerevan in 2015—competence featured in its widest range of reference: citizenship, lifelong employability, international mobility.

The Berlin formulation of 2003 spoke of a qualifications framework based on workload, level, learning outcomes, competences and profile, regarding learning outcomes and competences as different categories. It was historically significant, because it was in response to this ministerial communiqué that an informal joint Quality Initiative group developed the Dublin Descriptors in 2004.

The Descriptors set out the expected attributes of students who have successfully completed courses at short cycle, Bachelor, Master and doctoral levels. The term 'competence' is not used systematically; surprisingly, it appears only at Bachelor level, where it means that which may be appraised through the medium of the assessment process. Competence here has a retrospective reference—while the learning outcome has the prospective character of a result yet to be obtained.

The Bologna ministerial communiqués have a flavour all their own. They have to establish continuity between the summit meetings. They have also to express a unanimity which, given the rising number of signatory countries, tends to be couched in generalities rather than specifics. The growing emphasis on employability from 2005 onwards, in parallel with the policy statements of the EU, is clearly discernible, and yet a consecutive reading of all the communiqués yields an overwhelming sense of repetitiousness. Despite this, they provide no stable definition of competence.

Greater hopes might be placed in the Bologna Follow-Up Group (BFUG), which manages the Process on a self-regulatory basis in the intervals between the ministerial summits. BFUG includes stakeholder bodies capable of giving the debates a stronger bottom-up character and a greater potential to tap into the thinking of the higher education institutions, their staff and their students. Yet it, too, falls short of providing clear definition: 'learning outcomes are understood in their broadest sense and, in the case of the Dublin Descriptors and the Tuning project, include **competences**. Within some discourses, **competences** may have a more precise meaning, for example, in some assessment contexts they are associated with the performance of work-related tasks' [16] (p. 41).

In the Tuning project, meanwhile, competence reverts to the umbrella function that it enjoyed in the EU's Recommendation on Key Competences. Learning outcomes are subsumed within it, rather than standing apart as a separate category.

> **Competences** represent a combination of attributes (with respect to knowledge and its application, attitudes, skills and responsibilities) that describe the level or degree to which a person is capable of performing them. […] In this context, a **competence** or set of **competences** means that a person puts into play a certain capacity or skill and performs a task, where he/she is able to demonstrate that he/she can do so in a way that allows evaluation of the level of achievement. **Competences** can be carried out and assessed [17] (p. 69).

7. Competences in the European Credit Transfer and Accumulation System (ECTS)

ECTS was funded and developed on a pilot basis by the European Commission in the early years of the ERASMUS programme. Three versions of its Users' Guide have been published, the most recent of which (2015) was drafted by an ad hoc working group [18], chaired by the Commission but located within the framework of BFUG. What do the Users' Guides tell us of the nature of competence? [19].

The first edition in 2005 stuck close to the early Tuning position, presenting competences as bundles of attributes, while setting learning outcomes at a higher order of complexity—being sets of competences, or effectively bundles of bundles. The third edition (2015) reiterated the 2009 Glossary entry, reproducing the EQF definition, but adding a statement to the effect that 'learning outcomes express the level of competence attained by the student and verified by assessment' [20] (p. 22).

This assertion drew an immediate rebuttal from two of the most respected authorities on learning outcomes, Declan Kennedy and Marion McCarthy (both of University College Cork). They point out that there is a widely accepted definition of a learning outcome: a statement of what a learner is expected to know, understand and/or be able to demonstrate after completion of a process of learning, but 'there is no agreement' in the literature on the meaning of competence' [21] (p. 3). Indeed, they say, there is significant confusion, for which they hold the Tuning project responsible.

Kennedy and McCarthy recommend the EQF definition, re-stated below, because it is that which should apply to Common Training Frameworks developed in the framework of the amended Directive. It is therefore the definition which should be borne in mind by designers of competence-based curricula for sectoral professions.

> **Competence** means the proven ability to use knowledge, skills and personal, social and/or methodological abilities, in work or study situations and in professional and personal development. In the context of the European Qualifications Framework, **competence** is described in terms of responsibility and autonomy.

It is evident that it is easier to identify competences required in context than to unravel the epistemological and cognitive components of the concept of 'competence'.

This is, indeed, what pharmacists have done, as Antonio Sánchez Pozo has shown, writing in this collection of articles. They promote the competences deemed essential and desirable by professional consensus within their own scientific field. Their perception of competence derives from deontology, from the relevant knowledge base, and from the experience of professional practice. Their approach is principled and pragmatic. Rarely do they linger on definitions. Other criteria are more important: fulfilling prescribed ratios of theory to practice; satisfying the Competent Authorities that curricula are appropriate bases for registration; ensuring that the competences instilled in basic training can be clearly built upon and self-assessed in continuing professional development (CPD).

8. What Are the Next Steps in Competence-Based Curricula?

There remain high levels of graduate unemployment in numerous European countries [22] (pp. 182–208). Given that the bulk of students accessing higher education come directly from the secondary sector, there is also a need for renewed commitment to competence-based education in secondary education. This much was revealed by the 2015 report of the Programme of International Student Assessment (PISA). This was the first time that all EU MSs had participated simultaneously. The headline conclusion drawn by the European Commission makes dismal reading:

> When it comes to progress towards the 2020 benchmark of less than 15% low achievers, the EU as a whole is seriously lagging behind in all three domains and has taken a step backward, compared to the PISA 2012 results (science: 20.6%, +4.0 percentage points; reading: 19.7%, +1.9 percentage points; maths: 22.2%, +0.1 percentage point). Low achievers cannot successfully complete basic tasks that are required in modern societies and the consequences of this underachievement, if it is not tackled successfully, will be eminent and costly in the long run for them individually, but also for societies as a whole [23].

This unwelcome stimulus to policy-makers, with its negative implications for future higher education participation rates, concerns both those in the EU and those in the Bologna Process countries. Major policy shifts in the EU will be apparent by 2018, if they are to manifest themselves in programme opportunities in 2020. The next summit of the Bologna ministers is also scheduled for 2018, in Paris. What, at this stage, are their likely agendas?

In fact, the Commission has already adopted its *New Skills Agenda* [24]. It consists of ten actions to be implemented before the end of 2017. Most relevant to the present discussion are:

- a review of the Key Competences Recommendation, with a focus on skills acquired in non-formal and informal settings;
- a proposed Blueprint for sectoral cooperation on skills, which will identify skills gaps, assess their impact and develop strategies based on business-education partnerships; pilot work has already begun in six sectors, and the healthcare sector will follow later in 2017;
- a review of the EQF, designed to strengthen and broaden it, specifically by accelerating the process of referencing to it the national qualifications frameworks of EU and non-EU countries.

The review of the EQF has particular significance for pharmacists, as suggested in the final section of this article.

Much of the Commission's thinking is underpinned by the ambitious European Skills, Competences, Qualifications and Occupations venture (ESCO), which aims to map onto the EQF the detailed taxonomy of occupations developed by the International Labour Organisation (ILO). The outcome will be a fully-functioning multilingual website designed to facilitate 'competence-based job-matching'. Readers will be curious to discover the ESCO profile of pharmacy. It is a case of 'watch this space': the current online version is ESCO v0 [25], last updated in August 2014.

The ESCO planners may consider that it is of particular usefulness to the regulated professions. The truth of the matter could be the other way round: it is the professions, with their tabulations of competences in context, and their translations of competences into curricula, which can inform ESCO and higher education policy-makers.

The Commission has recognised that the demographic and socio-economic back-drop has changed significantly since the days of the Lisbon Strategy. A high-skilled labour force remains necessary, but this is now due to the probable displacement of millions of low-skilled occupations by automation and digital technologies. High-skilled job creation has become the order of the day; loss of social cohesion has become the greatest perceived risk.

In the Bologna Process, meanwhile, thoughts have turned to 'new policy goals' and a working group has been set up to carry this preoccupation forward. It is not wholly clear what will eventuate in the field of competences. It may be that the focus will shift back to citizenship, in the light of the advances made by resurgent nationalisms and parties of the extreme right. If this is the case, the Council of Europe's recent work on *competences for democratic culture* [26] will be a central feature.

Such a shift would act as a pendant to the EU's strong focus on labour market needs. The challenge for higher education systems and institutions would then be to find ways of implementing the two policy imperatives and of designing curricula which deliver both sets of competences in synergy.

The next review of the Directive is scheduled for 18 January 2019. Article 60.2 specifies that the review will report on, *inter alia*, 'the modernisation of the knowledge, skills and **competences** for the professions covered by Chapter III of Title III, [the seven sectoral professions] including the list of **competences** referred to in Article 31(7)' [general care nurses]; and 'the functioning of the common training frameworks and common training tests'.

9. Conclusions

In conclusion, it is useful to return to the proposed review [27] of the EQF. If the review proceeds as the Commission intends, its outcomes will figure in the next review of the Directive; they will emphatically confirm that EU higher education policy has primarily a labour market focus; and they will also therefore inflect discussions within BFUG.

What, then, is intended? If the Recommendation is adopted, it will:

- cover all qualifications, including private-sector, non-formal and international qualifications;
- develop a standard format for the expression of a learning outcome;

- attach learning outcomes to ECTS in a more systematic manner;
- include as many third country qualifications frameworks as possible;
- strengthen the governance of the EQF.

In respect of competence, it will take steps to enhance the clarity of its terminology. In its tabulation of levels, the word 'competence' will be replaced by 'responsibility and autonomy'. The next two years represent a window of opportunity for the pharmacists to finalise, implement and report on their competence-based curricula, in order to inflect positively any further amendments to the Directive and to impose their presence on higher education policy-makers.

Conflicts of Interest: The authors declare no conflict of interest.

Appendix A. Incidence of the Word 'Competence' in Bologna Ministerial Communiqués

Bologna 1999	A Europe of Knowledge is now widely recognised as an irreplaceable factor for social and human growth and as an indispensable component to consolidate and enrich the European citizenship, capable of giving its citizens the necessary **competences** to face the challenges of the new millennium, together with an awareness of shared values and belonging to a common social and cultural space.
Prague 2001	[no mention]
Berlin 2003	Ministers encourage the member States [i.e., the Bologna signatory countries] to elaborate a framework of comparable and compatible qualifications for their higher education systems, which should seek to describe qualifications in terms of workload, level, learning outcomes, **competences** and profile. They also undertake to elaborate an overarching framework of qualifications for the European Higher Education Area.
Bergen 2005	We adopt the overarching framework for qualifications in the EHEA, comprising three cycles (including, within national contexts, the possibility of intermediate qualifications), generic descriptors for each cycle based on learning outcomes and **competences**, and credit ranges in the first and second cycles. […] The European Higher Education Area is structured around three cycles, where each level has the function of preparing the student for the labour market, for further **competence** building and for active citizenship.
London 2007	Higher education should play a strong role in fostering social cohesion, reducing inequalities and raising the level of knowledge, skills and **competences** in society.
Leuven 2009	Student-centred learning and mobility will help students develop the **competences** they need in a changing labour market and will empower them to become active and responsible citizens. […] Lifelong learning involves obtaining qualifications, extending knowledge and understanding, gaining new skills and **competences** or enriching personal growth. […] With labour markets increasingly relying on higher skill levels and transversal **competences**, higher education should equip students with the advanced knowledge, skills and competences they need throughout their professional lives.
Budapest-Vienna 2010	We acknowledge the key role of the academic community—institutional leaders, teachers, researchers, administrative staff and students—in making the European Higher Education Area a reality, providing the learners with the opportunity to acquire knowledge, skills and **competences** furthering their careers and lives as democratic citizens as well as their personal development.

Bucharest 2012	Today's graduates need to combine transversal, multidisciplinary and innovation skills and **competences** with up-to-date subject-specific knowledge so as to be able to contribute to the wider needs of society and the labour market. […] Lifelong learning is one of the important factors in meeting the needs of a changing labour market, and higher education institutions play a central role in transferring knowledge and strengthening regional development, including by the continuous development of **competences** and reinforcement of knowledge alliances.
Yerevan 2015	Thanks to the Bologna reforms, progress has been made in enabling students and graduates to move within the EHEA with recognition of their qualifications and periods of study; study programmes provide graduates with the knowledge, skills and **competences** either to continue their studies or to enter the European labour market; institutions are becoming increasingly active in an international context; and academics cooperate in joint teaching and research programmes. […] By 2020 we are determined to achieve an EHEA where our common goals are implemented in all member countries to ensure trust in each other's higher education systems; where automatic recognition of qualifications has become a reality so that students and graduates can move easily throughout it; where higher education is contributing effectively to build inclusive societies, founded on democratic values and human rights; and where educational opportunities provide the **competences** and skills required for European citizenship, innovation and employment. […] Study programmes should enable students to develop the **competences** that can best satisfy personal aspirations and societal needs, through effective learning activities. […] We need to ensure that, at the end of each study cycle, graduates possess **competences** suitable for entry into the labour market which also enable them to develop the new **competences** they may need for their employability later in throughout their working lives. […] We will promote international mobility for study and placement as a powerful means to expand the range of **competences** and the work options for students. […]

Appendix B. Definitions of 'Competence' in Successive Editions of the ECTS Guide

ECTS Users' Guide 2005	Learning outcomes are sets of **competences**, expressing what the student will know, understand or be able to do after completion of a process of learning, long or short. […] **Competences** represent a dynamic combination of attributes, abilities and attitudes. […] **Competences** are formed in various course units and assessed at different stages. They may be divided in subject-area related competences (specific to a field of study) and generic competences (common to any degree course).

ECTS Guide 2009	In Europe a variety of terms relating to "learning outcomes" and "**competences**" are used with different shades of meaning and in somewhat different frames of reference. In all cases however they are related to what the learner will know, understand and be able to do at the end of a learning experience. [The] Guide cites the EQF definition of competence quoted earlier in this article, but goes on to provide the following further definition in its Glossary . . .] **Competence**: A dynamic combination of cognitive and metacognitive skills, knowledge and understanding, interpersonal, intellectual and practical skills, ethical values and attitudes. Fostering competences is the object of all educational programmes. Competences are developed in all course units and assessed at different stages of a programme. Some competences are subject-area related (specific to a field of study), others are generic (common to any degree course). It is normally the case that competence development proceeds in an integrated and cyclical manner throughout a programme.
ECTS Guide 2015	[The 2015 Guide retains the 2009 Glossary entry, itself based on the EQF definition of competence, but—in an attempt to disentangle competence from learning outcome—states that] . . . Learning outcomes express the level of **competence** attained by the student and verified by assessment.

References

1. Directive 2005/36/EC on the recognition of professional qualifications, now amended as Directive 2013/55/EU.
2. Corbett, A. *Universities and the Europe of Knowledge*; Palgrave Macmillan: London, UK, 2005.
3. Council of the European Union. *European Educational Policy Statements*; Supplement No. 2 to the Third Edition; Council of the European Communities General Secretariat: Luxembourg, 1993.
4. Study Group on Education and Training. *Accomplishing Europe through Education and Training*; Office for Official Publications of the European Communities: Luxembourg, 1997; p. 136.
5. Wim Kok (Group). *Facing the Challenge*; Wim Kok Report; Office for Official Publications of the European Communities: Luxembourg, 2004; Available online: https://ec.europa.eu/research/evaluations/pdf/archive/fp6-evidence-base/evaluation_studies_and_reports/evaluation_studies_and_reports_2004/the_lisbon_strategy_for_growth_and_employment__report_from_the_high_level_group.pdf (accessed on 25 March 2017).
6. Communication on Mobilising the Brainpower of Europe: Enabling Universities to Make Their Full Contribution to the Lisbon Strategy. 2005. Available online: http://eur-lex.europa.eu/legal-content/EN/TXT/PDF/?uri=CELEX:52005DC0152&from=EN (accessed on 25 March 2017).
7. Joint Interim Report on Education and Training 2010: The Success of the Lisbon Strategy Hinges on Urgent Reforms. 2004. Available online: http://register.consilium.europa.eu/doc/srv?l=EN&f=ST%206905%202004%20INIT (accessed on 25 March 2017).
8. All subsequent uses (including in Appendix A) of bold font for the word competence, when cited in extracts from published documents, are the author's emphases.
9. Recommendation 2006/962/EC on Key Competences for Lifelong Learning. Available online: http://eur-lex.europa.eu/legal-content/EN/TXT/PDF/?uri=CELEX:32006H0962&from=EN (accessed on 25 March 2017).
10. Recommendation on the Establishment of the European Qualifications Framework for Lifelong Learning. 2008. Available online: http://eur-lex.europa.eu/legal-content/EN/TXT/PDF/?uri=CELEX:32008H0506(01)&from=EN (accessed on 25 March 2017).
11. Authors of other articles in this collection address this question in much greater detail.
12. Council Directive 85/432/EEC of 16 September 1985 Concerning the Coordination of Provisions Laid Down by Law, Regulation or Administrative Action in Respect of Certain Activities in the Field of Pharmacy. Available online: http://eur-lex.europa.eu/LexUriServ/LexUriServ.do?uri=CELEX:31985L0432:EN:HTML (accessed on 25 March 2017).

13. Study on Transposition of the Directive on the Recognition of Professional Qualifications; Ramboll Consulting; Commissioned by the European Parliament Directorate General for Internal Policies. 2009, p. 65. Available online: http://www.europarl.europa.eu/document/activities/cont/200910/20091009ATT62184/20091009ATT62184EN.pdf (accessed on 25 March 2017).

14. For Full Details, see http://www.hospitalpharmacy.eu/how-the-project-is-progressing/ and, in particular, the presentation by Richard Price posted at http://www.eahp.eu/news/EU-monitor/eahp-eu-monitor-9-december-2016#overlay-context=news/EU-monitor (accessed 25 March 2017).

15. The extracts in which 'competence' appears are set out in Appendix A. The full text of each communiqué is available at http://www.ehea.info/pid34247/how-does-the-bologna-process-work.html (accessed on 25 March 2017).

16. Bologna Working Group on Qualifications Frameworks. *A Framework for Qualifications of the European Higher Education Area*; Ministry of Science, Technology and Innovation: Copenhagen, Denmark, 2005; p. 41. Available online: http://ufm.dk/en/publications/2005/a-framework-for-qualifications-of-the-european-higher-education-area (accessed on 25 March 2017).

17. González, J.; Wagenaar, R. *Tuning Educational Structures in Europe*; Final Report, Pilot Project—Phase 1; University of Deusto: Bilbao, Spain; University of Groningen: Groningen, The Netherlands, 2003; p. 69. Available online: http://www.bolognakg.net/doc/Tuning_phase1_full_document.pdf (accessed on 25 March 2017).

18. The present author was a member of the working group.

19. Their definitions of 'competence' are tabulated in Appendix B to this article.

20. *ECTS Users' Guide*; Publications Office of the European Union: Luxembourg, 2015; p. 22. Available online: http://ec.europa.eu/dgs/education_culture/repository/education/library/publications/2015/ects-users-guide_en.pdf (accessed on 25 March 2017).

21. Kennedy, D.; McCarthy, M. Learning Outcomes in the ECTS Users' Guide 2015. *J. Eur. High. Educ. Area* **2016**, 3. Available online: http://www.ehea-journal.eu/index.php?option=com_docman&task=doc_details&gid=432 (accessed on 25 March 2017).

22. European Commission/EACEA/Eurydice. *The European Higher Education Area in 2015: Bologna Process Implementation Report*; Publications Office of the European Union: Luxembourg, 2015; pp. 182–208. Available online: http://eacea.ec.europa.eu/education/eurydice/documents/thematic_reports/182EN.pdf (accessed on 25 March 2017).

23. PISA 2015: EU Performance and Initial Conclusions Regarding Education Policies in Europe. Available online: https://ec.europa.eu/education/sites/education/files/pisa-2015-eu-policy-note_en.pdf (accessed on 25 March 2017).

24. For the relevant documents, see http://ec.europa.eu/social/main.jsp?catId=1223&langId=en&moreDocuments=yes (accessed on 25 March 2017).

25. ESCO Portal. Available online: https://ec.europa.eu/esco/portal/browse (accessed on 25 March 2017).

26. Council of Europe. *Competences for Democratic Culture: Living Together as Equals in Culturally Diverse Democratic Societies*; Council of Europe: Strasbourg, France, 2016; Available online: http://www.coe.int/en/web/education/competences-for-democratic-culture (accessed on 25 March 2017).

27. Proposal for a Council Recommendation on the European Qualifications Framework for Lifelong Learning and Repealing the Recommendation of the European Parliament and of the Council of 23 April 2008 on the Establishment of the European Qualifications Framework for Lifelong Learning. Available online: https://ec.europa.eu/transparency/regdoc/rep/1/2016/EN/1-2016-383-EN-F1-1.PDF (accessed on 25 March 2017).

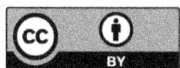

pharmacy

MDPI

Article

A Comparison of Competences for Healthcare Professions in Europe

Antonio Sánchez-Pozo

Department of Biochemistry, Faculty of Pharmacy, University of Granada, Campus Cartuja s/n, Granada 18071, Spain; sanchezpster@gmail.com; Tel.: +34-958-243-842

Academic Editor: Jeffrey Atkinson
Received: 5 December 2016; Accepted: 16 February 2017; Published: 21 February 2017

Abstract: In Europe and elsewhere, there is increasing interest in competence-based education (CBE) and training for professional practice in healthcare. This review presents competences for pharmacy practice in Europe and compares them with those for medicine and dentistry. Comparisons amongst competence frameworks were made by matching the European Directive for Professional Qualifications in sectoral professions such as healthcare (EU directive) with the frameworks of competences elaborated by European consortia in pharmacy (PHAR-QA), medicine (MEDINE), and dentistry (ADEE). The results show that the recommendations of the EU directive for all three professions are similar. There is also widespread similarity in the formulation of competences for all healthcare professions. Furthermore, for medicine and pharmacy, the rankings by practitioners of the vast majority of competences are similar. These results lay the foundations for the design of more interdisciplinary educational programs for healthcare professionals, and for the development of team-based care.

Keywords: competences; education; pharmacy; healthcare professions

---

1. Introduction

In Europe, and elsewhere in the world, there is an increasing shift from content-based to competence-based education (CBE) and practice. In healthcare sciences, this process started in medicine [1] and is now developing in pharmacy. This shift can bring many advantages. Competences for practice are better understood by the society at large, and thus provide a clearer public statement of the role of the healthcare practitioner. Competences are useful in the mutual recognition of qualifications amongst institutions and government bodies, especially at an international level as amongst European member states. CBE promotes greater comparability and compatibility in educational programs, thus facilitating student and practitioner mobility. The CBE approach also stimulates the development of advanced practice. In European pharmacy, CBE is at present limited; student [2] and practitioner mobility is low [3], and advanced practice, although developing, is still not recognized by the EU [4].

Competence frameworks for pharmacy education have emerged during the last years both at national, European, and worldwide levels. These have been promoted by professional chambers and associations, and academia [5–15]. European frameworks have been proposed for other healthcare sciences such as medicine (MEDINE: Medical education in Europe) [16] and dentistry (ADEE: Association for Dental Education in Europe) [17].

In this paper, we compared the CBE framework for EU pharmacies developed by the PHAR-QA (Quality assurance in European pharmacy education and training) [13] consortium (a follow-up to the PHARMINE (Pharmacy education in Europe) [14] project) with those for medicine (MEDINE [16]) and dentistry (ADEE [17]).

The comparison was carried out in three parts:

1. The recommendations for the minimum requirements of the EU directive [4].
2. The formulations of the academic proposals for CBE in healthcare sciences.
3. The perception by practitioners of the framework proposals for pharmacy and medicine. (This step has not to our knowledge been undertaken in dentistry).

EU Directives of the European Parliament and of the Council on the recognition of professional qualifications have consolidated a system of mutual recognition. It provides for automatic recognition for a limited number of professions based on harmonized minimum training requirements (sectoral professions), a general system for the recognition of evidence of training and automatic recognition of professional experience. The directives have also established a new system of the free provision of services.

Evaluation of the perception of practitioners is an essential step in building a framework. To do this, practitioners rank the competences proposed according to their own development needs, after reflection on the competences required for their particular professional practice. Faculties and other academic institutions have collaborated in the establishment of a framework of competences based on the scientific advances and new methodologies in education. Examples of this collaboration include the PHARMINE and MEDINE. However, the academic knowledge of the problems have to be tested in the working places. This dual approach—an academic proposal followed by ranking by practitioners—is an integral part of the production of a viable framework.

2. Results and Discussion

2.1. The Recommendations for Minimum Requirements of the European Directive

The 2013 EU directive on the recognition of professional qualifications [4], an amendment of the 2005 EU directive [18], deals mainly with structural management issues, such as length of degree course and the attributes of training, rather than competences. It does, however, set out a series of minimum requirements for the healthcare sciences (Table 1).

Table 1. The minimum requirements for healthcare professions as given in the 2005 EU directive [4].

Requirement	Pharmacy	Medicine	Dentistry
The sciences upon which practice is based	X	X	X
The scientific methods including the principles of measurement	X	X	X
Evaluation of scientific data	X	X	X
Structure, function and behavior of healthy and sick persons	X	X	X
Traineeship in a community or hospital setting	X	X	X
Clinical disciplines and practices		X	X

As shown in Table 1, the requirements of the EU directive for the sectoral professions of pharmacy, medicine (general practice), and dentistry have many things in common. Education and training for all three types of practitioner require basic science, human physiopathology, and clinical experience.

Only the requirements for medicine and dentistry, however, emphasize clinical disciplines in which the professional is in direct contact with healthy or sick individuals. However, there has been an evolution in pharmacy from the EU directive in its 2005 version [18] to its 2013 version [4] (Table 2), with the installation of a more "clinical" role for pharmacists as far as patient centered care and public health is concerned. Others professions such as nurses and midwives have also had changes in their requirements, whereas medicine and dentistry remain unchanged.

Table 2. Description of the roles of pharmacist given in the 2005 and 2013 EU directives. Differences in EU directives concerning patient care and public health issues are given in bold.

EU Directive 2005 [18]	EU Directive 2013 [4]
Preparation of the pharmaceutical form of medicinal products; manufacture and testing of medicinal products; testing of medicinal products in a laboratory for the testing of medicinal products; storage, preservation and distribution of medicinal products at the wholesale stage	Same as 2005
Preparation, testing, storage and supply of medicinal products in pharmacies open to the public	Ordering, manufacture, testing, storage and dispensing of safe, high quality medicinal products in public pharmacies
Preparation, testing, storage and dispensing of medicinal products in hospitals	Same as 2005
Provision of information and advice on medicinal products	Medication management and provision of information and advice about medicinal products and **general health information**
	Provision of advice and support to patients in connection with the use of non-prescription medicines and self-medication
	Contributions to public health and information campaigns

It should be noted that the elements given in Tables 1 and 2 are not competences. They describe knowledge or activities. For instance, the requirement "the sciences upon which practice is based" corresponds to the levels ("knows" and "knows how") of Miller's triangle [19]; or the "Provision of information and advice on medicinal products" corresponds to the levels ("shows how" and "does"). However, the EU directive still lacks detail on "competences for practice" and this is one of the reasons why the PHAR-QA, MEDINE, and ADEE academic consortia produced their detailed frameworks for pharmacy, medicine, and dentistry, respectively.

2.2. The Formulations of the Academic Proposals for CBE in Healthcare Sciences

A comparison was made of the competence frameworks proposed by academia for pharmacy (PHAR-QA), medicine (MEDINE), and dentistry (ADEE). The major competences were divided into domains as shown in Table 3. We grouped the competences in clusters of related competences: first in groups of very close competences that we called major competences, and then in domains of related major competences. For example, the major competence "professional attributes" includes competences such as probity, honesty, commitment to maintaining good practice, concern for quality, critical and self-critical abilities, reflective practice, and empathy, and the domain "professionalism" includes professional attributes, professional work, and ability to apply ethical and legal principles. This grouping facilitates comparisons, as the individual definitions of competences by the three consortia concerned are not always identical, even though they are talking about the same concept.

The following domains are common to all three professions: professionalism, interpersonal competences, communication and social skills, knowledge base, information and information literacy, clinical information gathering, diagnosis and treatment planning, therapy, establishing and maintaining health, and prevention and health.

The major competences included in the domains of Table 3 account for more than 95% of the major competences described in the frameworks. They can thus be considered as representative of the frameworks proposed.

Table 3. Domains and major competences in frameworks of competences for the pharmacist (PHAR-QA), general medical practitioner (MEDINE) and dentist (ADEE).

Domain	Major Competences		
	PHAR-QA	MEDINE	ADEE
1. Professionalism	Personal competences: values.	Professional attributes	Professional attitude and behavior
	Personal competences: learning and knowledge.	Professional working	
	Personal competences: values.	Apply ethical and legal principles	Ethics and jurisprudence
2. Interpersonal, communication and social skills	Personal competences: communication and organizational skills.	Communicate effectively in a medical context	Communication
3. Knowledge base, information and information literacy	Personal competences: learning and knowledge.	Apply the principles, skills and knowledge of evidence-based medicine	Application of basic biological, medical, technical and clinical sciences
	Personal competences: learning and knowledge.	Use information and information technology effectively in a medical context	Acquiring and using information
4. Clinical information gathering	Patient care competences: patient consultation and assessment.	Carry out a consultation with a patient	Obtaining and recording a complete history of the patient's medical, oral and dental state
		Assess psychological and social aspects of a patient's illness'	
5. Diagnosis and Treatment planning	Patient care competences: need for drug treatment.	Assess clinical presentations, order investigations, make differential diagnoses and negotiate a management plan	Decision-making, clinical reasoning and judgment
	Patient care competences: drug interactions.	Provide immediate care of medical emergencies, including First Aid and resuscitation'	
	Patient care competences: drug dose and formulation.		
	Patient care competences: provision of information and service.		
6. Therapy, establishing and maintaining health	Patient care competences: monitoring of drug therapy.	Carry out practical procedures	Establishing and maintaining oral health
		Prescribe drugs	
7. Prevention and health promotion	Patient care competences: patient education.	Promote health, engage with population health issues and work effectively in a health care system	Improving oral health of individuals, families and groups in the community

For each domain, peer major competences appear on the same line, whereas non-equivalent major competences appear on different lines (Table 3). There are gaps in the table (perhaps) representing major competences that (one or more) professions consider implicit.

The first three domains relate to personal competences and are very similar in all healthcare professions. A specific attitude and behavior to patients, together with an ethical commitment, are common aspects of these healthcare professions. Communication and social skills are clearly needed for the information and education of patients. As in many other professions, the use of information technology and the ability to solve problems is a common denominator.

The last four domains (4–7) comprise the specific competences related to patient care. Patient care requires (1) clinical judgment based on competences for gathering information included in the domain "Clinical information gathering"; (2) assessment and treatment planning, included in the domain "Diagnosis and Treatment planning"; and (3) monitoring the results, included in the domain "Therapy, establishing and maintaining health." These latter domains are present in all three healthcare professions. We suggest that the decisions about the need for a drug, the selection, dosage, the adverse effects, etc., typically performed by the pharmacist, follow the same principles as other clinical disciplines and thus require the same competences. This is reflected in the increasing role of pharmacists in patient care as recognized by the EU (see above).

2.3. The Perception by the Practitioners of the Framework Proposals for Pharmacy and Medicine

In the PHAR-QA [14] and MEDINE [16] projects the competences were ranked by practitioners in each profession.

Figure 1 shows that all competences were considered "necessary" (rank > 2/4), although with a considerable degree of variability. Globally, ranking scores for pharmacists and general practitioners were similar, although there were some differences. Knowledge of a second language and research skills were ranked higher by pharmacists; competences such as the ability to work autonomously and to recognize limits were ranked higher by general practitioners.

All patient care competences were considered "necessary" (rank >2/4) (Figure 2). The spread for patient care competences (2.9–3.8) was higher than for personal competences (2–3.8), suggesting that all practitioners rank patient care competences as more important. Rankings were similar for pharmacy and medicine with the global rank being lower for pharmacy than for medicine (delta = −0.5).

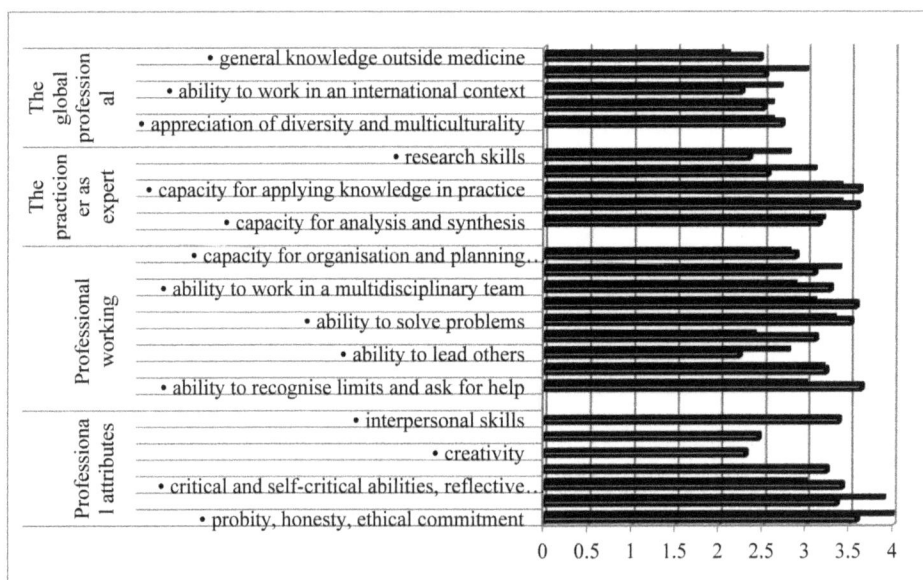

Figure 1. Ranking of personal competences by pharmacy (full columns) and medicine (open columns) practitioners. Ranking was on a 4-point scale (1 = least and 4 = most important). Pharmacy data are from PHAR-QA [19–22], and for medicine MEDINE [16].

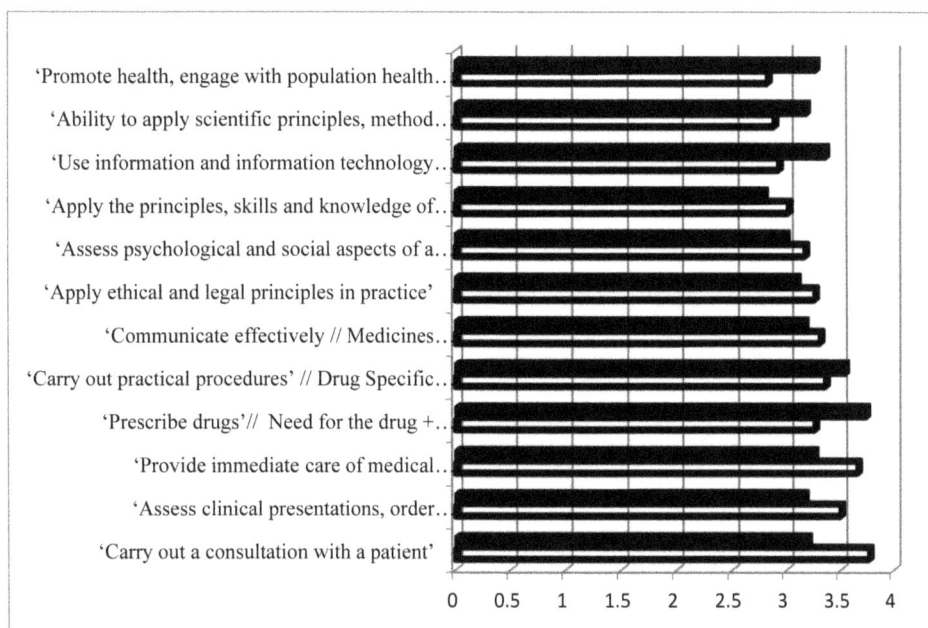

Figure 2. Ranking of patient care competences by pharmacy (full columns) and medicine (open columns) practitioners. Ranking was on a 4-point scale (1 = least and 4 = most important). Pharmacy data are from PHAR-QA [19–22], and for medicine MEDINE [16].

3. Conclusions

The results show that there is much similarity in competences for practice amongst all healthcare professions. This is seen in the recommendations for practice in the EU directive. It is also seen in the formulation of the competences by the different EU academic consortia that have proposed competence frameworks for pharmacy (PHAR-QA, medicine (MEDINE) and dentistry (ADEE)). Finally, it is seen in the perception of pharmaceutical and medical practitioners through their relative ranking of the proposals for competences.

The identification of a large number of competences that are similar in healthcare professions opens up the possibilities of a new design in educational programs with the installation of CBE, of more interaction in the different healthcare disciplines regarding education and practice, and, globally, of programs that are more adequate to an era of team-based healthcare.

Acknowledgments: I wish to thank J. Atkinson for his continuous help and support and for the revision of the manuscript. This work was supported by the Lifelong Learning program of the European Union: 527194-LLP-1-2012-1-BE-ERASMUS-EMCR.

Conflicts of Interest: The author declares no conflict of interest.

References

1. Frank, J.R.; Snell, L.S.; Cate, T.O.; Holmboe, E.S.; Carraccio, C.; Swing, S.R.; Harris, P.; Glasgow, N.J.; Campbell, C.; Dath, D.; et al. Competency-based medical education: Theory to practice. *Med. Teach.* **2010**, *32*, 638–645. [CrossRef] [PubMed]
2. Data on Intra-EU Student Mobility: Strengths and Diversity of European Student Mobility—Agence Erasmus. Available online: https://www.agence-erasmus.fr/docs/2115_soleoscope-10-en.pdf (accessed on 13 January 2017).

3. Wismar, M.; Maier, C.B.; Glinos, I.A.; Dussault, G.; Figueras, J. (Eds.) *Health Professional Mobility and Health Systems: Evidence from 17 European Countries*; Observatory Studies Series 23; WHO Regional Office for Europe on Behalf of the European Observatory on Health Systems and Policies: Copenhagen, Denmark, 2011. Available online: http://www.healthpolicyjrnl.com/article/S0168-8510(15)00214-6/fulltext#bibl0005 (accessed on 13 January 2017).

4. Directive 2013/55/EU of the European Parliament and of the Council of 20 November 2013 Amending Directive 2005/36/EC on the Recognition of Professional Qualifications and Regulation (EU) No 1024/2012 on Administrative Cooperation through the Internal Market Information System ('the IMI Regulation'). Available online: http://eur-lex.europa.eu/legal-content/EN/ALL/?uri=celex%3A32013L0055 (accessed on 13 January 2017).

5. General Level Framework. A Framework for Pharmacists Development in General Pharmacy Practice. Available online: http://www.codeg.org/fileadmin/codeg/pdf/glf/GLF_October_2007_Edition.pdf (accessed on 13 January 2017).

6. Core Competency Framework for Pharmacists. The Pharmaceutical Society of Ireland. Available online: http://www.thepsi.ie/gns/pharmacy-practice/core-competency-framework.aspx (accessed on 13 January 2017).

7. Competencias del Farmacéutico Para Desarrollar Los Servicios Farmacéuticos (SF) Basados en Atención Primaria de Salud (APS) y las Buenas Prácticas en Farmacia (BPF). Available online: http://forofarmaceuticodelasamericas.org/wp-content/uploads/2015/04/Competencias-del-farmacéutico-para-desarrollar-los-SF-basados-en-APS-y-BPF.pdf (accessed on 13 January 2017).

8. The American College of Clinical Pharmacy (ACCP). White Paper Clinical Pharmacist Competencies: The American College of Clinical Pharmacy. *Pharmacotherapy* **2008**, *28*, 806–815.

9. Medina, M.S.; Plaza, C.M.; Stowe, C.D.; Robinson, E.T.; DeLander, G.; Beck, D.E.; Melchert, R.B.; Supernaw, R.B.; Roche, V.F.; Gleason, B.L.; et al. Center for the Advancement of Pharmacy Education 2013 Educational Outcomes. *Am. J. Pharm. Educ.* **2013**, *77*, 162. [CrossRef] [PubMed]

10. Competency Framework for the Pharmacy Profession. Pharmacy Council of New Zealand, 2009. Available online: http://www.pharmacycouncil.org.nz/cms_show_download.php?id=201 (accessed on 13 January 2017).

11. NAPRA. Professional Competencies for Canadian Pharmacists at Entry to Practice. 2007. Available online: http://napra.ca/content_files/files/comp_for_cdn_pharmacists_at_entrytopractice_march2014_b.pdf (accessed on 13 January 2017).

12. National Competency Standards Framework for Pharmacists in Australia. Pharmaceutical Society of Australia, 2010. Available online: https://www.psa.org.au/downloads/standards/competency-standards-complete.pdf (accessed on 13 January 2017).

13. PHAR-QA (Quality Assurance in European Pharmacy Education and Training). 2016. Available online: http://www.phar-qa.eu/ (accessed on 13 January 2017).

14. The PHARMINE (Pharmacy Education in Europe) Consortium. Work Programme 3: Final Report. Identifying and Defining Competences for Pharmacists. Available online: http://www.pharmine.org/wp-content/uploads/2014/05/PHARMINE-WP3-Final-ReportDEF_LO.pdf (accessed on 13 January 2017).

15. A Global Competency Framework. FIP Pharmacy Education Taskforce, 2012. Available online: https://www.fip.org/files/fip/PharmacyEducation/GbCF_v1.pdf (accessed on 13 January 2017).

16. Learning Outcomes/Competences for Undergraduate Medical Education in Europe (MEDINE) the Tuning Project (Medicine). Available online: http://tuningacademy.org/medine-medicine/?lang=en (accessed on 13 January 2017).

17. Cowpe, J.; Plasschaert, A.; Harzer, W.; Vinkka-Puhakka, H.; Walmsley, A.D. Profile and Competences for the Graduating European Dentist—Update 2009. *Eur. J. Dent. Educ.* **2010**, *14*, 193–202. [CrossRef] [PubMed]

18. Directive 2005/36/EC of the European Parliament and of the Council of 7 September 2005 on the Recognition of Professional Qualifications. Available online: http://eur-lex.europa.eu/legal-content/EN/TXT/?uri=celex:32005L0036 (accessed on 15 February 2017).

19. Miller, G.E. The assessment of clinical skills/competences/performance. *Acad. Med.* **1990**, *65*, 63–67. [CrossRef]

20. Atkinson, J.; de Paepe, K.; Sánchez Pozo, A.; Rekkas, D.; Volmer, D.; Hirvonen, J.; Bozic, B.; Skowron, A.; Mircioiu, C.; Marcincal, A.; et al. How do European pharmacy students rank competences for practice? *Pharmacy* **2016**, *4*, 8. [CrossRef]

21. Atkinson, J.; de Paepe, K.; Sánchez Pozo, A.; Rekkas, D.; Volmer, D.; Hirvonen, J.; Bozic, B.; Skowron, A.; Mircioiu, C.; Marcincal, A.; et al. What is a pharmacist: Opinions of pharmacy department academics and community pharmacists on competences required for pharmacy practice. *Pharmacy* **2016**, *4*, 12. [CrossRef]

22. Atkinson, J.; Sánchez Pozo, A.; Rekkas, D.; Volmer, D.; Hirvonen, J.; Bozic, B.; Skowron, A.; Mircioiu, C.; Sandulovici, R.; Marcincal, A.; et al. Hospital and Community Pharmacists' Perceptions of Which Competences Are Important for Their Practice. *Pharmacy* **2016**, *4*, 21. [CrossRef]

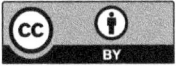

MDPI

Review
The Production of the PHAR-QA
Competence Framework [†]

Jeffrey Atkinson [1,2]

[1] Lorraine University, 5 rue Albert Lebrun, 54000 Nancy, France;
   jeffrey.atkinson@univ-lorraine.fr; Tel./Fax: +33-383-273-703
[2] Pharmacolor Consultants Nancy, 12 rue de Versigny, 54600 Villers, France
[†] This article is dedicated to the memory of Bartholomew Rombaut who passed away on the 23 January 2014.

Academic Editor: Yvonne Perrie
Received: 16 January 2017; Accepted: 27 March 2017; Published: 1 April 2017

Abstract: This article describes the background and methodology of the PHAR-QA (Quality Assurance in European Pharmacy Education and Training) project that produced a competence framework for pharmacy education and practice in the EU. In order to produce a harmonized competence framework that could be accepted within the EU situation, we developed a two-stage Delphi process centred on two expert panels. A small panel of academics produced the competence framework that was then validated by the rankings of a large panel consisting of representatives of the EU pharmacy community. The main aspects of this process are developed in this article.

Keywords: pharmacy; education; competences; framework; methodology

1. Introduction

This article describes the background and methodology of the PHAR-QA (Quality Assurance in European Pharmacy Education and Training) [1] project and provides several ideas on the methodology for those wishing to undertake a similar exercise. The results of the PHAR-QA have been published [2] and the reader of this article should refer to that paper for all details of the methodology, results, conclusions and perspectives.

PHAR-QA was planned to produce a competence framework for pharmacy education and training (PET) in Europe. It was a follow-up to the PHARMINE (Pharmacy Education in Europe) project [3] that surveyed the present situation of education and training in European pharmacy departments, both in terms of "structure" (resources and management, staff and student numbers, timing, duration of courses, subject areas taught, etc.), and "competences" (knowledge and ability to perform as pharmacy practitioners, quality assurance, etc.). Both projects took into account the wide diversity of pharmacy practice (community, hospital, industry, administrative, etc.) in the EU.

2. Background

2.1. Rationale: Why Carry Out the PHAR-QA Project

A first reason for considering the PHAR-QA project was the observation that European PET is extremely varied as far as structural aspects are concerned, and, furthermore, very little of it is based on competence learning [4]. The situation has not changed since the survey carried out by Pierre Bourlioux and the European Association of Faculties of Pharmacy, in the EU in 1994 [5].

The above situation is paradoxical in that there exists a European directive on the harmonization of the sectoral profession of pharmacy with recommendations for PET [6]. However, this—as all directives—is the result of the EU comitology process which tends to be aimed more towards resources and management rather than to ability. Thus, regarding PET, the EU directive focuses on 10 activities (e.g., "preparation of the pharmaceutical form") and 14 course subjects (e.g., "plant and animal biology"), with reference to wide competences (e.g., "adequate knowledge of medicines").

The above situation is unfortunate as one of the fundamental laws of the EU is the right of patients in the EU to efficient healthcare, regardless of the member state in which it is proffered. This is embedded in the EU directive on patients' rights to cross-border healthcare [7].

A second observation was that there is no harmonized European system for implementation and evaluation of competence-based learning and training in pharmacy [8]. In a survey on existing quality assurance and accreditation systems in 10 EU member states, we found that the existing schemes are based mainly on management and resources and little on competences. Furthermore, existing schemes are national and obligatory. Thus, in the EU, PET, as education and training in other sectors of healthcare, is organized on a confederal rather than a federal basis. A federal system assigns more power to the central government, whereas a confederate system reserves most of the power for the member states. This allows, therefore, substantial independence on the part of the member states regarding the way in which they organize PET in their specific country. Any attempt to impose a rigid, obligatory system for PET would probably fail given this European situation. This is why PHAR-QA proposed a harmonized, consultative system based not on management and resources but on competences. The ways in which pharmacy practice competences are gained will vary from one member state to another.

2.2. The Starting Points: Existing Competence Frameworks

In order to avoid the "NIH" ("not invented here") syndrome, a review of existing competence frameworks for PET, and those for education and training in other healthcare areas (medicine, dentistry, etc.), was carried out by A. Sanchez-Pozo and D. Rekkas (see chapter by A. Sanchez-Pozo in this special book edition). We also considered the recommendations outlined in the EU directive on the sectoral profession of pharmacy [6]. On the basis of the review, a list of proposed competences for pharmacy practice was produced.

3. Methodology

3.1. Type of Competence

Proposed competences were of two types: "knowledge/being aware of" and "ability/capable of doing". The first type of competence corresponds to the two lower levels ("knows/knowledge" and "knows how/competence") of Miller's triangle [9], the second to the two upper levels ("shows how/performance" and "does/action"). These two types of competences were proposed ("knowledge" and "ability") as the consortium considered that in some areas of pharmacy practice all students should be "aware of" without necessarily being "capable of doing". One example is "knowledge of design, synthesis, isolation, characterisation and biological evaluation of active substances". The consortium considered that students should be aware of such aspects of industrial pharmacy and R&D, without necessarily being capable of applying the methodology to synthesise, evaluate, etc., themselves. Competences were ranked on a 4-point ranking scale: from "not important/ can be ignored" to "essential/obligatory", proposed by the MEDINE (*Medical education in Europe*) consortium [10] with whom PHAR-QA collaborated.

3.2. The Two-Panel Delphi Process: The Small and Large Panels

The process used in the PHAR-QA project was a modified Delphi, two-stage process involving two panels: firstly, a small panel consisting of the 13 consortial members whose names and affiliations are given at the end of this article. All were academics with substantial experience in PET. The initial function of the small panel was to produce a questionnaire on the basis of the report on starting points (see Section 3.1. above). This was produced by three Delphi rounds. The second function of the small panel was to evaluate the results of the first round of the large panel Delphi (see below), and on the basis of this, to produce a second refined version for examination by the large panel. The large panel consisted of pharmacy students, academic staff and professionals (community, hospital, industrial pharmacists and pharmacists working in other fields). The large panel had two main functions: firstly, to rank the competences in two anonymous, Delphi rounds; secondly, to ensure the validation by the global pharmacy community of a competence framework produced by academics.

This large panel paradigm has been used but rarely in the production of competence frameworks in healthcare sciences; notable exceptions being the PHAR-QA project and MEDINE. As in MEDINE, it was used here in order to facilitate the acceptance of the final competence framework by both the professional community and university circles. This is a cardinal point in the PHAR-QA study. The major difference with MEDINE was that PHAR-QA ran two rounds of large panel ranking whereas MEDINE ran only one. This posed the question of the repeatability of the results using the PHAR-QA methodology (see Section 3.4 below).

3.3. Iteration versus Anonymity—Implications for the Repeatability of the Results

In order to ensure the anonymity of the respondents of the large panel, the option of collecting individual emails in the first round then using them in the second was not taken. The second round questionnaire was sent to the same email lists. Thus, iteration was maintained by sampling from the same population but not—intentionally—by contacting the same individuals.

The same individuals were probably contacted in the two rounds and some of them probably replied in the two rounds. The IT tool used automatically recorded the internet protocol (IP) address of the respondent computer. The survey also asked a number of questions on the respondent profile such as age category. Thus, double responders were identified as those with the same profile and the same IP number. There were between 5% and 16% of double responders in the different professional categories excepting students (0.6%).

3.4. Correlations between Results Obtained in the Two Delphi Rounds of the Large Panel

Figure 1 below shows the global rankings for the competences in rounds one and two. The ranking is very similar in the two rounds, showing that in spite of the fact that not exactly the same populations were questioned in the two rounds, the technique used—sampling from the same listings in the two rounds—allowed the confirmation of the rankings in the second round.

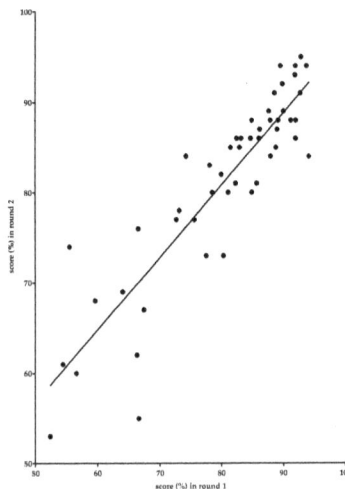

Figure 1. Global rankings of competences in the two rounds of the large panel Delphi process (for original see [2]).

The Spearman correlation between the scores in the two rounds was 0.881 ($p < 0.0001$).

3.5. Biases

One possible bias may arise from the use of English which is only one of the 24 official languages in the EU. In the United Kingdom and Ireland, more than 95% of the population understands English and in some Scandinavian countries, such as Sweden and Finland, half of the population understands English. However, in southern European countries such as Spain and Portugal, less than 15% understands English [11]. No data is available as to what percentage of pharmacists understands English in various European countries. Albeit, a plot of "number of responses" versus "capacity to speak English" (Figure 2) shows no relation between the two factors. This suggests that contributions from member states with a large percentage of the population capable of understanding English were not systematically greater than those from member states with a small percentage of the population capable of understanding English. In other words, it appears that the capacity to speak English did not introduce a bias in the conclusions drawn.

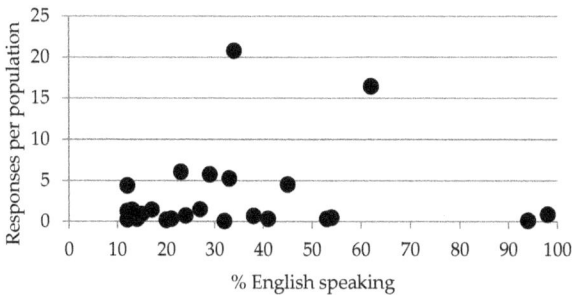

Figure 2. Number of respondents to the PHAR-QA (Quality Assurance in European Pharmacy Education and Training) survey in various countries versus the capacity of the population to speak English in the same country.

Responses per population = (total number of responses from pharmacy professionals (without students)/population of the country) × 1,000,000.

% English speaking = % of people in a given country who understand English well enough to follow the news on the radio or television [11].

Spearman correlation: 0.082 ($p > 0.05$).

Several strategies were used to minimize other biases. For instance, the small panel producing the survey to be examined by the large panel, examined the formulation of questions to avoid "leading questions" i.e., suggestive interrogation evoking a particular answer from a particular subgroup.

Other biases could have arisen from the way in which respondents were approached. In an attempt to avoid bias from partial "selected" responses, we sent the questionnaire to general populations of defined representative subgroups rather than to individuals. However, this by itself could have introduced a bias. The choice of the "representative subgroup" is crucial here. For instance, we used national student associations to contact students rather than sending the questionnaire to global listings of students, the latter being not always available in all countries. Thus, we harvested results from students motivated to join a student union. The counter argument here is that such students may well be the ones interested in change and evolution in PET. Furthermore, there may well be self-selection bias by respondents themselves with selection of those more concerned with the future of pharmacy. This may be desirable if the purpose of the Delphi procedure is to direct future developments rather than to confirm present opinions.

4. Conclusions and Perspectives

The main element of the PHAR-QA paradigm and methodology was the use of a two-panel ranking system to both establish a highly ranked competence framework, and to ensure the transfer of the latter to the end users i.e., the professional pharmacy community. This methodology is presented here with the objective of giving readers ideas as to the ways in which to produce competence frameworks.

Several perspectives are now open. Firstly, given the rapprochement of the different branches of healthcare education—for instance the introduction of the French PACES (première année commune aux études de santé or first year of healthcare studies)—it is becoming essential to produce a common competence framework for all-embracing healthcare education and practice.

Secondly, the pharmacy academic community needs to reflect on the ways in which competence frameworks could be introduced, starting with the matching of present degree courses to the competence framework.

Thirdly, the pharmacy professional community needs to reflect on how competence training can be applied in the workplace and how the professional community can interact with the academic world. One interesting aspect of this is the development of the validation of experiential learning in pharmacy. This is important in terms of the potential validation of the work experience of pharmacy technicians wishing to pursue a degree course in pharmacy. It is also important in the validation of practical experience of pharmacy students in those parts of the world where PET does not rigidly follow the model developed in Europe.

Acknowledgments: With the support of the Lifelong Learning program of the European Union: 527194-LLP-1-2012-1-BE-ERASMUS-EMCR. This project was funded with support from the European Commission. This publication reflects the views only of the author; the Commission cannot be held responsible for any use which may be made of the information contained therein.

Author Contributions: Jeffrey Atkinson wrote the first and subsequent revised versions of this article. The views expressed are those of the author; those of the individual members of the PHAR-QA consortium may be different.

Conflicts of Interest: The author declares no conflicts of interest.

Abbreviations

PET   pharmacy education and training
EU   European Union

Appendix A

On behalf of the PHAR-QA (Quality Assurance in European Pharmacy Education and Training) consortium:

1. Jeffrey Atkinson, Pharmacology Department, Lorraine University, 5 rue Albert Lebrun, 54000 Nancy, and Pharmacolor Consultants Nancy, 12 rue de Versigny, 54600 Villers, France; Jeffrey.atkinson@univ-lorraine.fr.
2. Kristien De Paepe, Pharmacy Faculty, Vrije Universiteit Brussel, Laarbeeklaan 103, Brussels 1090, Belgium; kdepaepe@vub.ac.be. Kristien De Paepe replaced Bartholomew Rombaut who passed away on the 23 January 2014.
3. Antonio Sánchez Pozo, Faculty of Pharmacy, University of Granada, Campus Universitario de la Cartuja s/n, Granada 18701, Spain; sanchezpster@ugr.com.
4. Dimitrios Rekkas, School of Pharmacy, National and Kapodistrian University Athens, Panepistimiou 30, Athens 10679, Greece; rekkas@pharm.uoa.gr.
5. Daisy Volmer, Pharmacy Faculty, University of Tartu, Nooruse 1, Tartu 50411, Estonia; daisy.volmer@ut.ee.
6. Jouni Hirvonen, Pharmacy Faculty, University of Helsinki, Yliopistonkatu 4, P.O. Box 33-4, Helsinki 00014, Finland; jouni.hirvonen@helsinki.fi.
7. Borut Bozic, Faculty of Pharmacy, University of Ljubljana, Askerceva cesta 7, Ljubljana 1000, Slovenia; Borut.Bozic@ffa.uni-lj.si.
8. Agnieska Skowron, Pharmacy Faculty, Jagiellonian University, Golebia 24, Krakow 31-007, Poland; askowron@cm-uj.krakow.pl.
9. Constantin Mircioiu, Pharmacy Faculty, University of Medicine and Pharmacy "Carol Davila" Bucharest, Dionisie Lupu 37, Bucharest 020021, Romania; constantin.mircioiu@yahoo.com.
10. Annie Marcincal, Faculty of Pharmacy, European Association of Faculties of Pharmacy, Université de Lille 2, Lille 59000, France; annie.marcincal@pharma.univ-lille2.fr.

11. Andries Koster, Department of Pharmaceutical Sciences, European Association of Faculties of Pharmacy, Utrecht University, PO Box 80082, 3508 TB Utrecht, The Netherlands; A.S.Koster@uu.nl.
12. Keith Wilson, School of Life and Health Sciences, Aston University, Birmingham B47ET, UK; k.a.wilson@aston.ac.uk.
13. Chris van Schravendijk, Medical Faculty, Vrije Universiteit Brussel, Laarbeeklaan 103, 1090 Brussels, Belgium; chris.Van.Schravendijk@telenet.be.
14. Lea Noel, Pharmacy Faculty, Vrije Universiteit Brussel, Laarbeeklaan 103, 1090 Brussels, Belgium; Lea.Noel@vub.ac.be (consortial secretary).

With the assistance of:

1. Richard Price, the European Hospital Pharmacists' Association. Available online: http://www.eahp.eu/ (accessed on13 January 2017).
2. Jamie Wilkinson, the Pharmacists' Group of the European Union. Available online: http://www.pgeu.eu/ fr/accueil.html (accessed on13 January 2017).
3. Jane Nicholson, European Industrial Pharmacists' Group. Available online: http://eipg.eu/ (accessed on 13 January 2017).
4. The President, European Pharmacy Students' Association, Available online: http://eafponline.eu/ (accessed on 13 January 2017).
5. The President, European Association of Faculties of Pharmacy. Available online: http://eafponline.eu/ (accessed on 13 January 2017).

References

1. The PHAR-QA Project. Quality Assurance in European Pharmacy Education and Training. Available online: www.phar-qa.eu (accessed on 13 January 2017).
2. Atkinson, J.; de Paepe, K.; Sánchez Pozo, A.; Rekkas, D.; Volmer, D.; Hirvonen, J.; Bozic, B.; Skowron, A.; Mircioiu, C.; Marcincal, A.; et al. The Second Round of the PHAR-QA Survey of Competences for Pharmacy Practice. *Pharmacy* **2016**, *4*, 27. [CrossRef]
3. The PHARMINE (Pharmacy Education in Europe) Consortium. Work Programme 3: Final Report Identifying and Defining Competences for Pharmacists. Available online: http://www.pharmine.org/wp-content/ uploads/2014/05/PHARMINE-WP3-Final-ReportDEF_LO.pdf (accessed on 13 January 2017).
4. Atkinson, J. Heterogeneity of Pharmacy Education in Europe. *Pharmacy* **2014**, *2*, 231–243. [CrossRef]
5. Bourlioux, P. Second European Meeting of the Faculties, Schools and Institutes of Pharmacy, Berlin, Germany, 27–28 September 1994.
6. The EU Directive 2013/55/EU on the Recognition of Professional Qualifications. Available online: http://eur-lex.europa.eu/LexUriServ/LexUriServ.do?uri=OJ:L:2005:255:0022:0142:EN:PDF (accessed on 13 January 2017).
7. The EU Directive 2011/24/EU on Patients' Rights in Cross-border Healthcare. Available online: http://ec.europa.eu/health/cross_border_care/towards_legislative_framework/index_en.htm (accessed on 13 January 2017).
8. Atkinson, J.; Rombaut, B.; Sánchez Pozo, A.; Rekkas, D.; Veski, P.; Hirvonen, J.; Bozic, B.; Skowron, A.; Mircioiu, C.; Marcincal, A.; et al. Systems for Quality Assurance in Pharmacy Education and Training in the European Union. *Pharmacy* **2014**, *2*, 17–26. [CrossRef]
9. Miller, G.E. The assessment of clinical skills/competences/performance. *Acad. Med.* **1990**, *65*, 63–67. [CrossRef]
10. MEDINE: Medical Education in Europe. MEDINE Is Concerned with the Mobility of Medical Students and Practitioners, the Standards and Content of Medical Education Programmes, the Transparency and Comparability of Qualifications, the Application of the Bologna Principles to Medical Education, and the Application of Medical Research to Education. Available online: http://medine2.com/Public/about.html (accessed on 13 January 2017).
11. Europeans and Their Languages. "Special Eurobarometer 386" of the European Commission (2012). Available online: ec.europa.eu/public_opinion/archives/ebs/ebs_386_en.pdf (accessed on 13 January 2017).

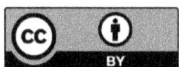

pharmacy

MDPI

Article

A Comparison of Parametric and Non-Parametric Methods Applied to a Likert Scale

Constantin Mircioiu [1] and Jeffrey Atkinson [2,*]

[1] Pharmacy Faculty, University of Medicine and Pharmacy "Carol Davila" Bucharest, Dionisie Lupu 37, Bucharest 020021, Romania; constantin.mircioiu@yahoo.com

[2] Pharmacolor Consultants Nancy, 12 rue de Versigny, Villers 54600, France

* Correspondence: jeffrey.atkinson@univ-lorraine.fr

Academic Editor: Nick Shaw

Received: 13 January 2017; Accepted: 8 May 2017; Published: 10 May 2017

Abstract: A trenchant and passionate dispute over the use of parametric versus non-parametric methods for the analysis of Likert scale ordinal data has raged for the past eight decades. The answer is not a simple "yes" or "no" but is related to hypotheses, objectives, risks, and paradigms. In this paper, we took a pragmatic approach. We applied both types of methods to the analysis of actual Likert data on responses from different professional subgroups of European pharmacists regarding competencies for practice. Results obtained show that with "large" (>15) numbers of responses and similar (but clearly not normal) distributions from different subgroups, parametric and non-parametric analyses give in almost all cases the same significant or non-significant results for inter-subgroup comparisons. Parametric methods were more discriminant in the cases of non-similar conclusions. Considering that the largest differences in opinions occurred in the upper part of the 4-point Likert scale (ranks 3 "very important" and 4 "essential"), a "score analysis" based on this part of the data was undertaken. This transformation of the ordinal Likert data into binary scores produced a graphical representation that was visually easier to understand as differences were accentuated. In conclusion, in this case of Likert ordinal data with high response rates, restraining the analysis to non-parametric methods leads to a loss of information. The addition of parametric methods, graphical analysis, analysis of subsets, and transformation of data leads to more in-depth analyses.

Keywords: ranking; Likert; parametric; non-parametric; scores

---

1. Introduction

Statistical methods have the following as prime functions: (1) the design of hypotheses and of experimental procedures and the collection of data; (2) the synthetic presentation of data for easy, clear, and meaningful understanding; and (3) the analysis of quantitative data to provide valid conclusions on the phenomena observed. For these three main functions, two types of methods are usually applied: parametric and non-parametric. Parametric methods are based on a normal or Gaussian distribution, characterized by the mean and the standard deviation. The distribution of results is symmetric around the mean, with 95% of the results within two standard deviations of the mean. Nonparametric statistics are not based on such parameterized probability distributions or indeed on any assumptions about the probability distribution of the data. Parametric statistics are used with continuous, interval data that shows equality of intervals or differences. Non-parametric methods are applied to ordinal data, such as Likert scale data [1] involving the determination of "larger" or "smaller," i.e., the ranking of data [2].

Discussion on whether parametric statistics can be used in a valid, robust fashion for the presentation and analysis of non-parametric data has been going on for decades [3–6]. Theoretical simulations using computer-generated data have suggested that the effects of the non-normality of distributions, unequal variances, unequal sample size, etc. on the robustness of parametric methods are not determinant [7], except in cases of very unusual distributions with a low number of data.

Regarding ordinal Likert data, the theoretical discussion of "parametric versus non-parametric" analysis continues [8,9]. In this paper, we will investigate this from a practical angle using real Likert data obtained in a recent study on pharmacy practitioners' ranking of competencies required for pharmacy practice [10]. The differences and similarities amongst the different subgroups of pharmacists are discussed in detail in the latter paper. In this paper, we ask a specific question on statistical methodology: does the significance of the differences within and amongst subgroups of practitioners in the rankings of the importance of competencies for practice diverge with the type of analysis (parametric or non-parametric) used? We will use the data for community pharmacists and their comparison with those for industrial pharmacists as an example.

The history behind the choice of dataset for this article is as follows. The PHAR-QA project had as primary endpoint the estimation of the core competencies for pharmacy graduate students that are by and large accepted by all subgroups whatever the statistical method used; this is presented in the results section. The secondary end-point consisted in the differences between professional subgroups and we found clear differences between groups whatever the statistical method used. As is suggested by the significance of the interaction term, these differences amongst subgroups are largely centered on particular competencies (see results). This paper follows those already published on this PHAR-QA survey, and its primary purpose is to compare the use and conclusions of parametric and non-parametric analyses.

2. Experimental Section

The data analyzed were from an on-line survey involving 4 subgroups of respondents:

1. community pharmacists (CP, $n = 183$),
2. hospital pharmacists (HP, $n = 188$),
3. industrial pharmacists (IP, $n = 93$), and
4. pharmacists in other occupations (regulatory affairs, consultancy, wholesale, ..., OP, $n = 72$).

Respondents were asked to rank 50 competencies for practice on a 4-point Likert scale:

1 = Not important = Can be ignored.
2 = Quite important =Valuable but not obligatory.
3 = Very important = Obligatory (with exceptions depending upon field of pharmacy practice).
4 = Essential = Obligatory.

There was a "cannot rank" check box as well as a possibility of choosing not to rank at all (blank). The questionnaire response rate was calculated as the distribution between "cannot rank + choose not to rank" versus "rank (1 + 2 + 3 + 4)."

Analysis was carried out on the numbers of values for each of the 4 ranks for each of the 50 competencies. Data were also transformed into binary scores = obligatory/total% = (numbers of values for Ranks 3 and 4)/total number of values for ranks, as a percentage [11]. Such transformation leads to a loss of information but a gain in granularity and in understanding.

Results are presented in three sections starting with reflections on the distribution of the data. This is followed by a section of parametric and non-parametric presentation of the data and a final section on parametric and non-parametric analyses of the data. Data were analyzed using GraphPad software [12] and in-house Excel spreadsheets.

3. Results and Discussion

3.1. Distribution of the Data

The questionnaire response rate between "cannot rank + choose not to rank" versus "rank" was globally 14.5:85.5 ($n = 536$ respondents); there were no significant differences in response rate amongst the four subgroups (chi-square, $p > 0.05$). This aspect was not pursued further given that the vast majority of respondents (86%) were able to understand and reply to the 50 questions on competencies. It can be inferred that differences in distributions of ranking values were not based on misunderstanding of questions.

There were no differences amongst subgroups in the response rate for individual competencies (= number of responses/50) (chi-square, $p > 0.05$). Missing values were not replaced.

The distributions of the ranking data are shown in Figure 1.

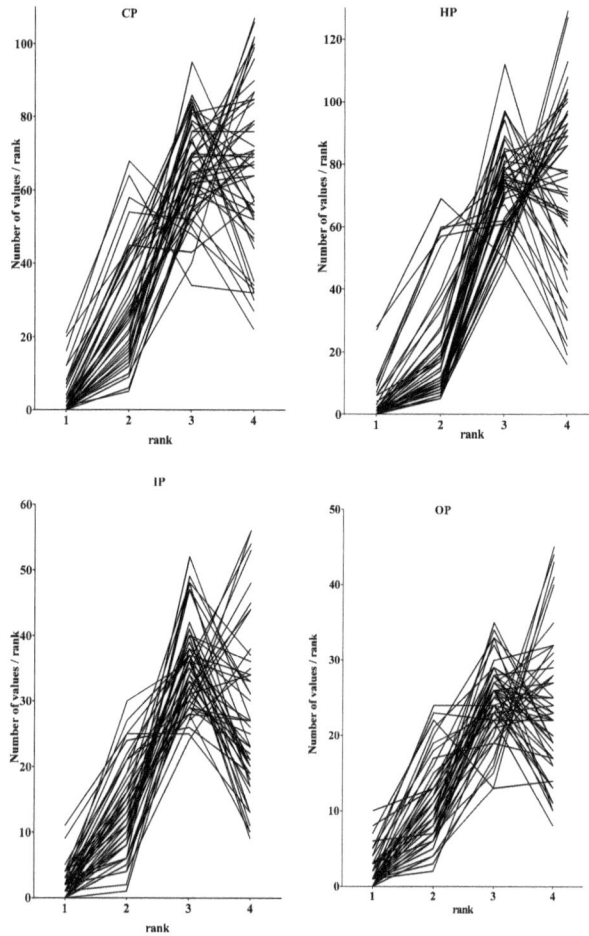

Figure 1. Distributions of ranking data (number of values/rank) for each of the 50 ranked competencies (lines). The four subgroups are as follows: community pharmacists (CP, $n = 183$ respondents, top left); hospital pharmacists (HP, $n = 188$, top right); industrial pharmacists (IP, $n = 93$, bottom right); pharmacists in other occupations such as regulatory affairs, consultancy, and wholesale (OP, $n = 72$, bottom left).

Visual inspection of the four graphs reveals that there were no outliers. Distributions visually suggested a non-Gaussian distribution, i.e., neither continuous nor bell-shaped. Given the small numbers of bins involved ($n = 4$ ranks), tests of normality of distribution such as the Kolmogorov–Smirnov test were not performed.

Distributions were, however, very similar in all four subgroups. They were of two types: inverted "j" or "linear/exponential"; both types of distribution were skewed to the left, i.e., to higher ranking values (on the right of each graph). In order to estimate the numbers of each type of distribution in individual subgroups of pharmacists, the "inverted j" was defined as having a negative value for "number of values for Rank 4–number of values for Rank 3", and the "linear/exponential" was defined as having a positive value for Rank 4–Rank 3.

The "inverted j" distribution was defined as having a negative value for "number of values for Rank 4–number of values for Rank 3", and the "linear/exponential" distribution was defined as having a positive value for "number of values for Rank 4–number of values for Rank 3."

Table 1 shows the numbers of "inverted j" and "linear/exponential" distributions. Chi-square analysis showed a difference between IP and the other three subgroups ($p < 0.05$). This is also seen in the visual inspection of the graphical representation in Figure 1. Distributions of negative and positive values were normal in all four subgroups; means of values "Rank 4–Rank 3" were not different from zero ($p > 0.05$).

Figure 2 contains the values for the differences in "number of values for Rank 4–number of values for Rank 3" for 50 competencies in the four subgroups. There were two clusters of negative values for competencies 13–30 and 38–50, indicating distributions of the "inverted j" form and two clusters of positive values for competencies 1–13 and 31–37, indicating "linear/exponential" distributions of ranking data. Thus, although sample distributions of ranks within competencies are not normal, they are similar in form from one competency to another, and one subgroup of pharmacists to another.

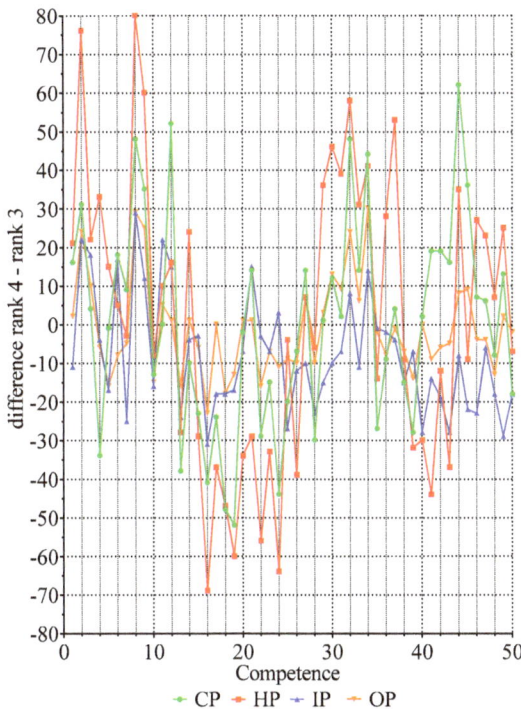

Figure 2. Values for the difference Rank 4–Rank 3 for all four subgroups. The four subgroups are as follows: community pharmacists (CP, n = 183 respondents, green circles); hospital pharmacists (HP, n = 188, red squares); industrial pharmacists (IP, n = 93, blue triangles); pharmacists in other occupations such as regulatory affairs, consultancy, and wholesale (OP, n = 72, orange inverted triangles).

Table 1. Numbers of negative and positive values for "number of values for Rank 4–number of values for Rank 3", range, means, standard deviations, and Kolmogorov–Smirnov test for normality, in the four subgroups of pharmacists.

Subgroup	CP	HP	IP	OP
Numbers of inverted j distributions	24	25	39	28
Numbers of linear/exponential distributions	26	25	11	22
Mean of values Rank 4–Rank 3	0.2	1.6	−7.7	−1.1
Standard deviation	27	37	15	12
Kolmogorov–Smirnov (KS) normality test				
KS distance	0.085	0.11	0.12	0.12
Passed normality test (alpha = 0.05)?	Yes	Yes	Yes	Yes

The situation here is one of similar distributions with different numbers of values (ranging from 72 for OP to 188 for HP). Boneau [7], using simulated data, found that, if numbers were large enough (>15), such a situation should not be problematic in terms of parametric analysis. Below, we shall determine whether this statement applies to the actual data.

3.2. Presentation and Analysis of Within-Subgroup Data

The question asked here is as follows: Within a given subgroup (CP will be used as an example), are there significant differences amongst the 50 competencies?

Graphic presentations of the medians, means, and scores of data for the ranking of the 50 competencies by CP, HP, IP, and OP are given in Figure 3.

For CP, whichever form of graphical presentation is used, the major features were the same, namely, that competencies 2, 8, 9, 12, 27, 32, 34, 42, 44, and 45 were ranked higher, and competencies 20 and 39 lower, than the others. The graphs for means and scores visually suggest that there may be significant differences amongst the other 38 competencies as more discriminant information is gathered by the use of parametric statistics (means) and data transformation (scores).

Although somewhat skewed to the right, the distributions of the means and scores were not significantly different from normal (Shapiro–Wilk and Kolmogorov–Smirnov test, $p < 0.05$). The number of bins was too small to test the distribution of medians (Figure 4).

To test for significant differences amongst rankings for comparisons between competencies across subgroups, we used (1) parametric 1-way ANOVA followed by the Bonferroni multiple comparisons test and (2) non-parametric Kruskal–Wallis analysis followed by the Dunn multiple comparisons test. Both analyses showed that there was a significant effect of "competency" (Table 2); both analyses gave the same very low *p*-values.

There were 8095 data points analyzed with 1055 missing values (11.5% of total (= 50 × 183 = 9150)). Missing values were not replaced.

Table 2. Parametric (top) and non-parametric (bottom) analyses of the significance of the effect of competency using the ranking data for CP ($n = 183$).

		Parametric			
1-Way ANOVA	**Sum of Squares**	**Degrees of Freedom**	**Mean Square**	**F (49, 8045)**	***p*-Value**
Treatment (competencies)	611.2	49	12.47	22.99	$p < 0.0001$
Residual	4365	8045	0.5426		
Total	4976	8094			
		Non-Parametric			
		Kruskal–Wallis Test			
	p-value (for competencies)				<0.0001
	Kruskal–Wallis statistic				720.8

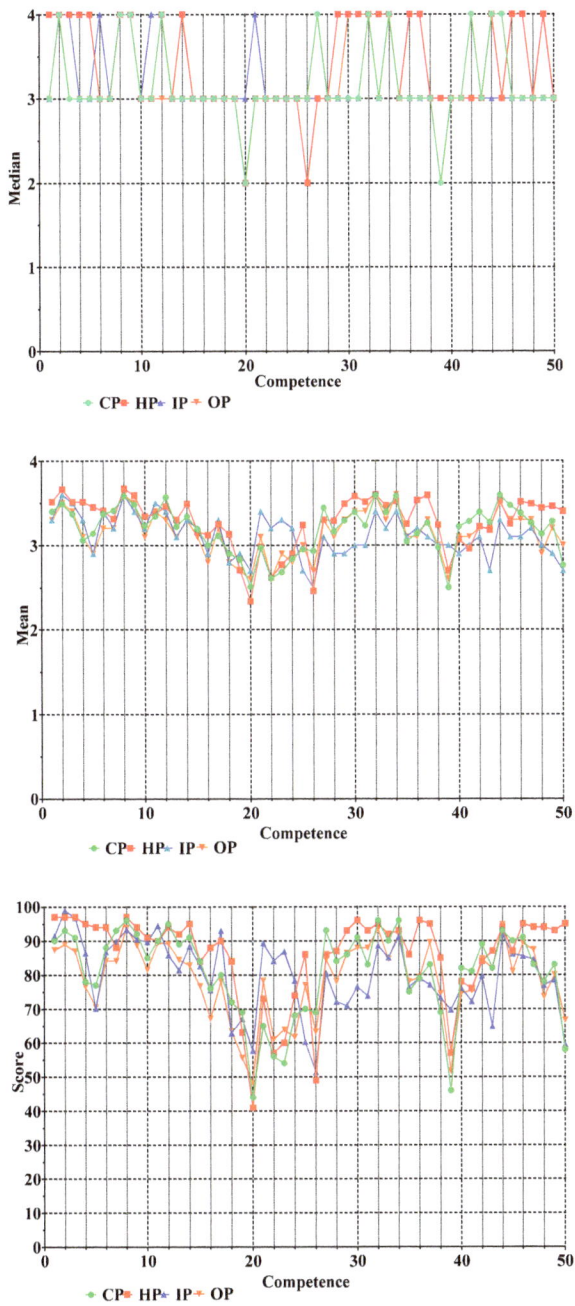

Figure 3. Graphic presentation of the data for the ranking of the 50 competencies. The four subgroups are as follows: community pharmacists (CP, *n* = 183 respondents, green circles), hospital pharmacists (HP, *n* = 188, red squares), industrial pharmacists (IP, *n* = 93, blue triangles), and pharmacists in other occupations such as regulatory affairs, consultancy, and wholesale (OP, *n* = 72, orange inverted triangles).

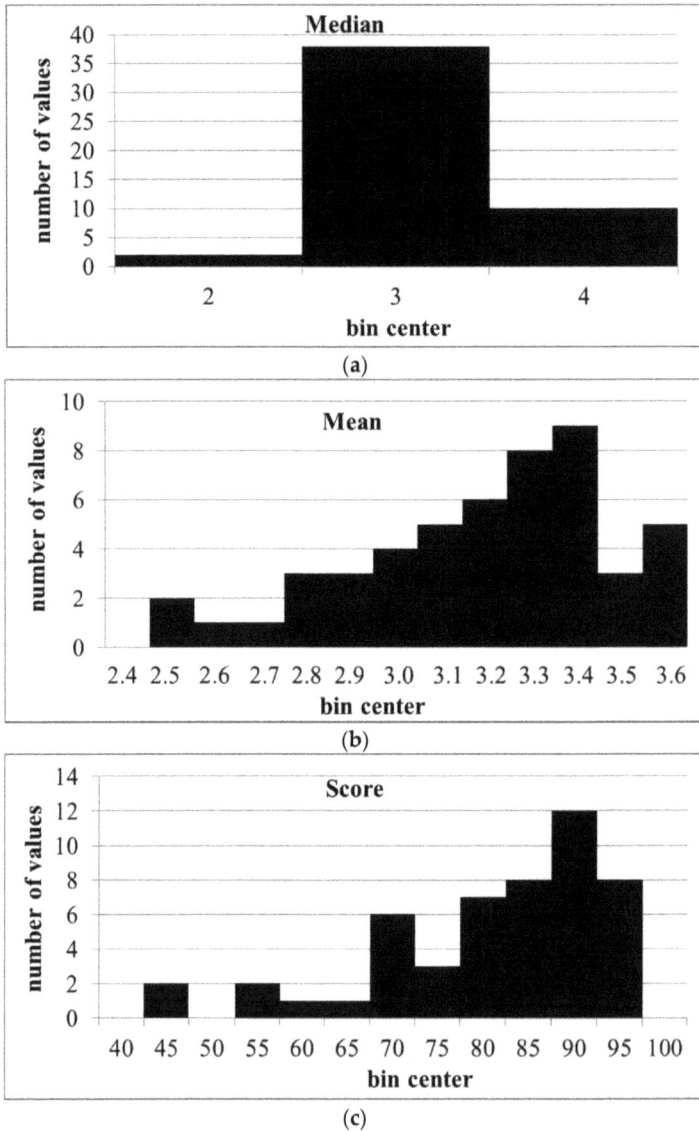

Figure 4. Distributions of medians, means, and scores of ranks for competencies given by CP (same data as in Figure 3). (**a**): medians; (**b**): means; (**c**): scores.

The total number of possible multiple comparisons amongst the 50 competencies was 1225. There was agreement between the parametric and non-parametric tests in the case of a conclusion of "not significant" (756 cases) (Table 3). The Bonferroni test revealed a significant difference in 469/1225 = 38% of the comparisons. There was disagreement between the parametric Bonferroni test and the non-parametric Dunn test in 76 (6%) of these cases, the Bonferroni producing a significant result but not the Dunn test (Table 3).

Table 3. Comparison of the significance of the differences amongst rankings for competencies within subgroups obtained by the parametric Bonferroni and the non-parametric Dunn tests (data for CP).

		Dunn	Dunn	
		Significant	Not significant	Total
Bonferroni	Significant	393	76	469
Bonferroni	Not significant	0	756	756
	Total	393	832	1225

The similarity of difference of competency-ranking (Table 3) by parametric and non-parametric methods can be formally assessed by the kappa test [13].

In this case, P_o = (proportion of observed agreement) = 0.94 and P_r = (proportion of random agreement) = 0.54.

$$\kappa = \frac{p_o - p_r}{1 - p_r} = 0.86$$

As we obtained a value 0.86, this can be considered as very good agreement.

In summary, both tests revealed significant and non-significant differences. In the majority of cases, the tests indicated the same result. The parametric Bonferroni test detected more significant differences than the non-parametric Dunn test, showing that the parametric test was more discriminate.

3.3. Presentation and Analysis of Amongst-Subgroup Data

The question asked was as follows: Are there significant differences between subgroups for one or several of the 50 competencies?

Figure 3 (above) shows the ranking data for the four subgroups in the form of medians (upper), means (middle), and scores (lower). Differences amongst subgroups are difficult to see in the case of medians. Means reveal granularity in results for the different subgroups. This shows, for example, that results for competencies 21–23 and 28–30 as ranked by IP (triangles) appear different from those of the other subgroups such as CP (circles). Such differences are accentuated in the graph of scores.

Individual ranking data for each competency in each subgroup were analyzed using a parametric two-way ANOVA with Sidak's multiple comparisons test, and the non-parametric Friedman test with Dunn's multiple comparisons test analyses (Table 4), in order to determine differences amongst subgroups.

The parametric two-way ANOVA revealed a significant effect of competency, subgroup, and the interaction "subgroup–competency" (Table 4). The percentage variation for competency was much greater than that for subgroup, suggesting that global differences amongst competencies were much greater than those amongst subgroups. Sidak's multiple comparisons test (Table 4) showed a significant difference between CP and IP or OP. Although the interaction "subgroup–competency" is highly significant, this type of analysis does not permit any conclusion as to which specific competencies are significantly different between two given subgroups (this will be dealt with later using the parametric multiple *t*-test and the non-parametric chi-square test). It could be argued that the interaction effect (F-value = 3.6) could be a spurious consequence of the relatively large primary competency effect (F-value = 38). We consider that the interaction effect is not spurious. The interaction effect is real since there are special clusters of competencies that are ranked differently in different professional subgroups (see Figure 3, e.g., CP versus IP for competencies 21–23).

Table 4. Parametric (upper) and non-parametric (lower) analyses of ranking data for four subgroups of pharmacists. (**a**) Parametric two-way ANOVA and Sidak's multiple comparisons test for differences amongst subgroups (number of missing values: 14,328). (**b**) Non-parametric Friedman analysis with Dunn's multiple comparisons test for differences amongst subgroups.

(a)

ANOVA Table	Sum of Squares	% of Total Variation	Degrees of Freedom	Mean Square	F	*p*
Interaction: competency–subgroup	289	2.1	147	2.0	$F_{(147, 22,872)} = 3.6$	$p < 0.0001$
Competency	1032	7.3	49	21	$F_{(49, 22,872)} = 38$	$p < 0.0001$
Subgroup	17	0.12	3	5.7	$F_{(3, 22,872)} = 10$	$p < 0.0001$
Residual	12,517		22,872	0.55		

Sidak's Multiple Comparisons Test, Comparisons with CP Only Are Given	Difference of Means	95% Confidence Limits of Difference	*p*-Value Summary
CP versus HP	0.0087	−0.019 to 0.036	Not significant
CP versus IP	0.0630	0.029 to 0.098	$p < 0.0001$
CP versus OP	0.0520	0.014 to 0.090	$p < 0.01$

(b)

	Friedman Statistic					10.05
	p-value					0.0182
	Number of subgroups					4

Dunn's Multiple Comparisons Test, Comparisons with CP Only Are Given	Rank Sum 1	Rank Sum 2	Sum Difference	N1	N2	*p*
CP versus HP	139.0	139.0	0.0	50	50	$p > 0.05$
CP versus IP	139.0	106.0	33.00	50	50	$p > 0.05$
CP versus OP	139.0	116.0	23.00	50	50	$p > 0.05$

The large number of missing values in this two-way ANOVA (38% of total) emphasizes the unbalanced nature of the analysis with numbers per subgroup ranging from 188 (HP) to 72 (OP). This can often occur in real-life surveys.

Non-parametric Friedman analysis (Table 4) also revealed a significant overall effect of subgroup, but Dunn's multiple comparisons test failed to reveal any significant effect of any specific combination of subgroup. It was thus less discriminant than Sidak's parametric multiple comparisons test. Furthermore, the Friedman test does not allow for the evaluation of the significance of interactions and so again provides less information than the two-way ANOVA.

Differences in specific competencies between two given subgroups were analyzed using the parametric multiple *t*-test and the non-parametric chi-square test. Amongst the multitude of potential combinations, data are shown (Table 5) for the comparisons between CP and IP for the six competencies revealed in Figure 3 above.

Table 5. Comparison of the chi-square test with the parametric *t*-test for the differences in competencies between CP and IP. For both tests, all values are $p < 0.05$.

Competency	*t*-Test	Chi-Square
21	3.49	17.2
22	4.99	22.9
23	5.18	27.9
28	2.93	10.4
29	3.63	13.7
30	3.47	12.1

In this example, it can be seen that the use of a parametric or a non-parametric test leads to the same conclusion regarding statistical significance (Table 5). As can be observed in Figure 5, the correlation between the *t*-test and chi-square test is good and approximately linear.

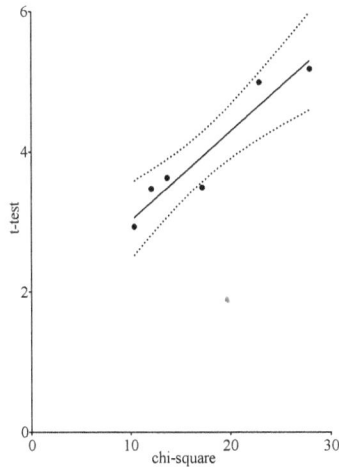

Figure 5. Correlation between the chi-square test and *t*-test for the competencies given in Table 5 in the comparison CP versus IP. (*t*-test = ((0.13 × chi-square) + 1.73), r^2 = 0.91).

4. Conclusions

Likert data from an actual survey are neither continuous nor Gaussian in distribution, and numbers per subgroup vary widely. In spite of this, parametric analyses are "robust" [14] as judged from the observation that parametric and non-parametric analyses lead to similar conclusions regarding statistical significance. The explanation for this may lie in the fact that numbers are large and distributions are similar.

Graphical representation in the form of scores provided an easier visual appreciation of differences. The calculation of scores, however, leads to a loss of information as a 4-point Likert scale is transformed into a binary scale. We suggest that this could be "compensated" by determining the difference between scores on the basis of a non-parametric chi-square test on the original ranking data.

Applying parametric analysis of real survey data leads practically in all cases to the same conclusions as those drawn from applying non-parametric analyses. Thus, the advantages of parametric analysis [15], which as seen above is more discriminant, can be exploited in a robust fashion. Several authors have criticized this position and argued on theoretical grounds that parametric analysis of ordinal data such as Likert rankings is inappropriate [4]. Others, after extensive analysis, have reached different conclusions. Thus, Glass et al. [16] concluded that "the flight to non-parametrics was unnecessary principally because researchers asked 'are normal theory ANOVA assumptions met?' instead of 'how important are the inevitable violations of normal theory ANOVA assumptions?'" In this paper, we have attempted to follow the same pragmatic approach. Likewise, Norman [9], after dissecting the argument that parametric analysis cannot be used for ordinal Likert scales, reached the conclusion that "parametric statistics are robust with respect to violations of these assumptions parametric methods can be utilized without concern for 'getting the wrong answer.'" Finally, Carifio and Perla [17], after considering the arguments, counter-arguments and empirical evidence found "many persistent claims and myths about 'Likert scales' to be factually incorrect and untrue."

In the light of the above, we suggest that, in the case presented here, the use of scores for graphical representation plus chi-square for analysis of Likert data, which (1) facilitates the visual appreciation of the data and (2) avoids the futile "parametric" versus "non-parametric" debate, assured the best mosaic of statistical tests combined with phenomenological analysis.

In our example, sample sizes are large (=/>72) and the question can be asked as to how sample size could affect our conclusions. It is certain that, according to the laws of large numbers, experimental frequencies tend in probability to theoretical probability, but the rapidity of such convergence was not our aim. The problem of sample size was discussed by Boneau [7], who suggested that "samples of sizes of 15 are generally sufficient to undo most of the damage inflicted by violation of assumptions. Only in extreme cases involving distributions differing in skew [authors' note: as was the case in our example] would it seem that slightly larger sizes are prescribed say, 30, for extreme violations." It should be noted, however, as discussed by Norman [9], that, "Nowhere is there any evidence that non-parametric tests are more appropriate than parametric tests when sample sizes get smaller." Curtis et al. argued—on theoretical grounds—that (more or less equal) numbers per group is also an important factor for ensuring robustness of statistical analysis [18]. Again, in our pragmatic approach, sample sizes varying from 72 to 188 did not appear to affect the issue.

Another possible issue concerns homogeneity of variance given that the IP data show some differences in distribution to those of the other three subgroups. This does not seem to be a problem given the similarities between the parametric and non-parametric analyses of CP versus IP. This is in agreement with the work of Boneau [7], on simulated data, who concluded "that for a large number of different situations confronting the researcher, the use of the ordinary t test and its associated table will result in probability statements which are accurate to a high degree, even though the assumptions of homogeneity of variance and normality of the underlying distributions are untenable. This large number of situations has the following general characteristics: (a) the two sample sizes are equal or nearly so (authors' note: this was not the case in our example); (b) the assumed underlying population distributions are of the same shape or nearly so."

Acknowledgments: With the support of the Lifelong Learning programme of the European Union: 527194-LLP-1-2012-1-BE-ERASMUS-EMCR. This project has been funded with support from the European Commission. This publication reflects the views only of the author; the Commission cannot be held responsible for any use that may be made of the information contained therein.

Author Contributions: J.A. and C.M. conceived the project; J.A. made the initial calculations and analyses; these were then checked by C.M., who suggested further analyses; J.A. wrote the manuscript that was corrected by C.M.; J.A. and C.M. participated equally in the revision of the manuscript.

Conflicts of Interest: The authors declare no conflict of interest.

References

1. Likert, R. A technique for the measurement of attitudes. *Arch. Psychol.* **1932**, *22*, 5–55.
2. Stevens, S.S. On the theory of scales of measurement. *Science* **1946**, *103*, 677–680. [CrossRef] [PubMed]
3. Feinstein, A.R. *Clinical Biostatistics. Chapter 16: On Exorcising the Ghost of Gauss and the Curse of Kelvin*; Mosby: Saint Louis, MO, USA, 1977.
4. Kuzon, W.M.; Urbanchek, M.G.; McCabe, S. The seven deadly sins of statistical analysis. *Ann. Plast. Surg.* **1996**, *37*, 265–272. [CrossRef] [PubMed]
5. Knapp, T.R. Treating ordinal scales as interval scales: An attempt to resolve the controversy. *Nurs. Res.* **1990**, *39*, 121–123. [CrossRef] [PubMed]
6. Gardner, P.L. Scales and statistics. *Rev. Educ. Res.* **1975**, *45*, 43–57. [CrossRef]
7. Boneau, C.A. The effects of violations of assumptions underlying the *t*-test. *Psychol. Bull.* **1960**, *57*, 49–64. [CrossRef] [PubMed]
8. Jamieson, S. Likert scales; how to (ab)use them. *Med. Educ.* **2004**, *38*, 1212–1218. [CrossRef] [PubMed]
9. Norman, G. Likert scales, levels of measurement and the "laws" of statistics. *Adv. Health Sci. Educ.* **2010**, *15*, 625–632. [CrossRef] [PubMed]
10. Atkinson, J.; De Paepe, K.; Sánchez Pozo, A.; Rekkas, D.; Volmer, D.; Hirvonen, J.; Bozic, B.; Skowron, A.; Mircioiu, C.; Marcincal, A.; et al. The PHAR-QA Project: Competence Framework for Pharmacy Practice—First Steps. The Results of the European Network Delphi Round 1. *Pharmacy* **2015**, *3*, 307–329. [CrossRef]
11. Marz, R.; Dekker, F.W.; van Schravendijk, C.; O'Flynn, S.; Ross, M.T. Tuning research competencies for Bologna three cycles in medicine: Report of a MEDINE2 European consensus survey. *Perspect. Med. Educ.* **2013**, *2*, 181–195. [CrossRef] [PubMed]

12. GraphPad Prism 7 for Biostatistics, Curve Fitting and Scientific Graphing. 2017. Available online: https://www.graphpad.com/ (accessed on 10 January 2017).
13. Landis, J.R.; Koch, G.G. The measurement of observer agreement for categorical data. *Biometrics* **1977**, *33*, 159–174. [CrossRef] [PubMed]
14. Box, G.E.P. Non-normality and tests on variances. *Biometrika* **1953**, *40*, 318–335. [CrossRef]
15. Gaito, J. Non-parametric methods in psychological research. *Psychol. Rep.* **1959**, *5*, 115–125. [CrossRef]
16. Glass, G.V.; Peckham, P.D.; Sanders, J.R. Consequences of Failure to Meet Assumptions Underlying the Fixed Effects Analyses of Variance and Covariance. *Rev. Educ. Res.* **1972**, *42*, 237–288. [CrossRef]
17. Carifio, J.C.; Perla, R.J. Ten Common Misunderstandings, Misconceptions, Persistent Myths and Urban Legends about Likert Scales and Likert Response Formats and their Antidotes. *J. Soc. Sci.* **2007**, *3*, 106–116. [CrossRef]
18. Curtis, M.J.; Bond, R.A.; Spina, D.; Ahluwalia, A.; Alexander, S.P.A.; Giembycz, M.A.; Gilchrist, A.; Hoyer, D.; Insel, P.A.; Izzo, A.A.; et al. Experimental design and analysis and their reporting: New guidance for publication in BJP. *Br. J. Pharmacol.* **2015**, *172*, 3461–3471. [CrossRef] [PubMed]

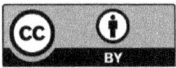

Article

Competence-Based Pharmacy Education in the University of Helsinki

Nina Katajavuori, Outi Salminen, Katariina Vuorensola, Helena Huhtala, Pia Vuorela and Jouni Hirvonen *

Faculty of Pharmacy, University of Helsinki, P.O. Box 56, 00014 Helsinki, Finland;
nina.katajavuori@helsinki.fi (K.N.); outi.salminen@helsinki.fi (S.O.); katariina.vuorensola@helsinki.fi (V.K.);
helena.huhtala@helsinki.fi (H.H.); pia.vuorela@helsinki.fi (V.P.)
* Correspondence: jouni.hirvonen@helsinki.fi

Academic Editor: Jeffrey Atkinson
Received: 16 January 2017; Accepted: 17 May 2017; Published: 1 June 2017

Abstract: In order to meet the expectations to act as an expert in the health care profession, it is of utmost importance that pharmacy education creates knowledge and skills needed in today's working life. Thus, the planning of the curriculum should be based on relevant and up-to-date learning outcomes. In the University of Helsinki, a university wide curriculum reform called 'the Big Wheel' was launched in 2015. After the reform, the basic degrees of the university are two-cycle (Bachelor–Master) and competence-based, where the learning outcomes form a solid basis for the curriculum goals and implementation. In the Faculty of Pharmacy, this curriculum reform was conducted in two phases during 2012–2016. The construction of the curriculum was based on the most relevant learning outcomes concerning working life via high quality first (Bachelor of Science in Pharmacy) and second (Master of Science in Pharmacy) cycle degree programs. The reform was kicked off by interviewing all the relevant stakeholders: students, teachers, and pharmacists/experts in all the working life sectors of pharmacy. Based on these interviews, the intended learning outcomes of the Pharmacy degree programs were defined including both subject/contents-related and generic skills. The curriculum design was based on the principles of constructive alignment and new structures and methods were applied in order to foster the implementation of the learning outcomes. During the process, it became evident that a competence-based curriculum can be created only in close co-operation with the stakeholders, including teachers and students. Well-structured and facilitated co-operation amongst the teachers enabled the development of many new and innovative teaching practices. The European Union funded PHAR-QA project provided, at the same time, a highly relevant framework to compare the curriculum development in Helsinki against Europe-wide definitions of competences and learning outcomes in pharmacy education.

Keywords: curriculum; learning outcomes; competency; stakeholders; generic skills

1. Introduction

In order to meet the expectations of an expert in the health care profession, it is of utmost importance that pharmacy education also creates the knowledge and skills needed in working life and to serve society. Pharmacists are in responsible positions within the health care system and therefore high quality, competence-based pharmacy education is needed [1–5].

Competence can be defined as a specialized system of abilities, proficiencies, or skills that are necessary to reach a specific goal. The term also refers to special functional competencies which are needed in a particular area of expertise [6]. In competence-based curriculum, four features are emphasized: focus on outcomes, emphasis on abilities, a reduced emphasis on time-based training and learner centeredness [7]. Thus, a competence-based curriculum in higher education aims at responding to the needs of the working life. In a competence-based curriculum the defined learning outcomes describe what the students are expected to know, understand and/or be able to do after completing a degree or in order to attain a passing grade in a course [8]. The definition of the learning outcomes take into account not only the expertise in the field, but also the knowledge and skills required for employment [9]. Furthermore, the discipline's latest developments and trends, as well as the changing learning needs and requirements of employers, need to be taken account [10].

The defined learning outcomes describe the knowledge, skills, and attitudes thought to be essential for a professional individual in their working life [11]. It is possible to divide the competencies into three categories: (1) Discipline-specific knowledge and skills; (2) Generic knowledge and skills for knowledge work; and (3) Knowledge and skills related to the expert identity (e.g., [10,12]). Carefully defined learning outcomes should aid the students to better understand what kind of knowledge and skills are needed in their profession after graduation and to direct their learning during (and after) their studies, and thus, aid the students to study more effectively and in a deep-level manner [8].

Learning outcomes should be defined for the whole study programs in the University, but also for each study-module and individual course within the program. Thus, the defined learning outcomes are more general at the program level, and more specified in the module and course levels ([8] Biggs & Tang 2011). The defined learning outcomes for the program affect both the curriculum design and teaching. The curriculum structure, as well as the teaching methods, should be derived from and linked to the specified learning objectives [2,8,13]. Furthermore, the assessment should be criterion-based and should validly be related to learning outcomes. John Biggs [2,13] coined the term "constructive alignment" to describe this kind of high quality curriculum design. In a constructively aligned curriculum the learning outcomes, course contents, teaching methods, and assessment are aligned and foster students' deep-level learning. In other words, constructive alignment highlights the importance of applying the defined competencies and learning outcomes to real-life teaching practices throughout the curriculum.

An extensive education reform, called 'the Big Wheel', was launched at the University of Helsinki in 2015. The aim of this reform is to create competence-based curricula with defined learning outcomes for all the study programs in the University in order to equip the students with the most relevant knowledge and skills needed in today's working life. In addition, the reform aims at producing the most qualified programs, education, and teaching practices throughout the University in order to foster the students' deep-level learning via the constructive alignment. Each study program (Bachelor and Master) has a degree program director and a steering group to ensure the quality of the programs. The competence-based teaching in the multidisciplinary programs makes it possible for a student to reach the ability to "think big", to perceive the whole picture and to assess connections in different contexts. There is also an increasing need to develop broadly such skills as critical thinking, information analysis, and communication (see [5,9,10]).

Faculty of Pharmacy, University of Helsinki, offers Bachelor's, Master's, and Doctoral Degree programs in pharmacy education. Students complete the Bachelor's Degree (180 credits) in three years and Master's Degree (additional 120 credits) in five years. The studies include a compulsory 3 + 3 month work practice in a community and/or hospital pharmacy during their second and third study-years. The majority of the graduating students find a job in community pharmacies, followed by hospital pharmacies, drug industry and research, education, and administration.

In the Faculty of Pharmacy, the curriculum reform was launched already in 2012, before the Big Wheel reform of the entire University of Helsinki commenced. There was a true need to define the competencies and to create learning outcomes for the Bachelor's and Master's programs in Pharmacy. The teachers, students, and employers all pointed out the need to update teaching contents and practices according to the rapidly developing knowledge and practices in various fields of pharmacy profession. These renewals in Helsinki can be directly related to and compared with the process and outcomes of the PHAR-QA project. This article summarizes these developmental activities and is focused on the processes of the reforms as well as on the outcomes.

2. Process of the Curriculum Reform

The learning outcomes for both the Bachelor's and Master's degree programs were created during 2012–2016. In addition, contents and practices of teaching were reformed to meet the intended learning outcomes in order to follow the principles of constructive alignment [3,8,13]. The curriculum reform took place in two phases: the first (2012–2014) focused on the Bachelor's program and the second (2015–2017) on the Master's program. Both the renewals were conducted by a named team, which consisted of senior lecturers in pharmacy education, a senior lecturer in higher education, and a member of administrative staff. The teams cooperated closely with the Educational Committee of the Faculty and organized several hearings and interviews for all the professors, teachers, and students in the Faculty.

In the beginning of the reform, the team carefully studied all the relevant information about the recent evaluations and research reports of pharmacy education and study subjects together with feedback from curriculum and course evaluations. In addition, the team benchmarked exemplary educational units on health care and management in order to find out the best practices for conducting the educational reform. Based on this familiarization, specific aims for the curriculum reform were formed: (1) to create the learning outcomes for the Bachelor's and Master's programs which would meet the needs of working life; (2) to create a more challenging curriculum and to develop teaching and assessing methods which would foster students' deep level learning and active work by students; and (3) to increase the flexibility of the curriculum and the amount of optional studies and thereby strengthen the professional orientation and identity of the students.

In order to define the learning outcomes, the team arranged hearings for all the relevant parties in autumn 2012. The needs of the working life representatives were found out by interviewing a broad sample of stakeholders in the field of pharmacy. For example, community and hospital pharmacies, the pharmaceutical industry, and authorities in the pharmacy sector were interviewed. The team interviewed also faculty teachers in each discipline, pharmacy students, and international staff of the faculty. The interviews were conducted as focus group discussions. In each interview, there were three to nine participants and they lasted for 60–120 min. Furthermore, all the professors of the faculty were interviewed individually in order to hear their visions in more detail and to engage them to the reform. More than 30 interviews were performed with 83 interviewees altogether.

The interviews explored the competencies, knowledge, and skills a pharmacy student should gain by graduation in order to excel in working life in the field of pharmacy. Detailed notes were written during every interview and the notes written were visible to all the participants in the discussions. The notes were commented on and corrected during the discussion if needed. The data of the interviews was analyzed by content analysis method by grouping and categorizing similar themes. In spring 2013, based on the analyses, the team formulated a draft of the learning outcomes including both subject/contents knowledge and generic skills for the Bachelor's and Master's programs (see [9,10]). The learning outcomes were further developed, defined, and finalized in several workshops during the spring and autumn 2013. All the interviewed stakeholders, teachers, and students of the faculty were invited to these workshops. The aims of the workshops were to inform about the process and also to discuss important and current themes which rose up from the interviews or from the process. In this respect, the process resembled the iterative character of the Delphi methodology in the PHAR-QA project. Also, the next steps in the reform were decided upon together in the workshops (Figure 1).

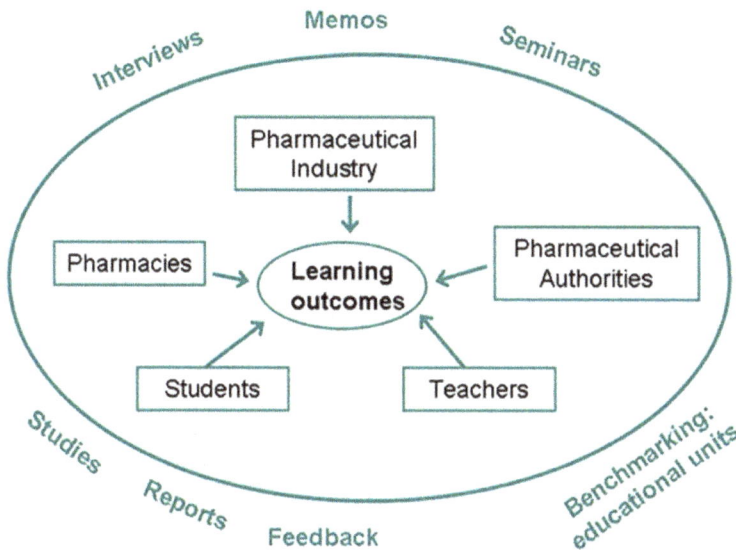

Figure 1. Defining the learning outcomes for Bachelor's and Master's programs in pharmacy.

3. The Outcomes of the Curriculum Reform

Formation of the new curriculum was a communal process between the University and working life. The curriculum, its contents, and the learning outcomes for the degree programs were discussed and processed together with teachers, stakeholders, and students (see [3,8]). The atmosphere during the process was enthusiastic and allowed everyone to participate in the process. An increased and systematic co-operation between the university teachers was grounded during the curriculum reform process in order to foster communal learning (e.g., [14,15]). As a result, many of the new practices developed during the curriculum reform were created in longitudinal processes in close co-operation with teachers. In addition, closer co-operation between the university teachers and the stakeholders was established.

3.1. The Learning Outcomes

The learning outcomes for the programs were defined and, for the first time, the learning outcomes for the programs in pharmacy education in Helsinki also included generic skills (Table 1). When the learning outcomes are defined for the program-level, they are at a more general level. More detailed learning outcomes should be defined at module and course levels of the program [8]. Importance of generic skills in working life were highly emphasized in the interviews. Although the backgrounds of the interviewees were quite different, the learning outcomes proposed by different stakeholders were surprisingly uniform. In addition to critical thinking and problem solving skills, the importance of professionalism rose up in the interviews. Pharmacy students should develop their professional identity during the studies. That includes the importance of realizing one's role in a health care system and understanding the significance and versatility of the pharmacy field. The core of the pharmaceutical knowledge was, however, to be focused on drug(s) and medication and the education should give a strong basis for this pharmaceutical knowledge and expertise. Defined generic learning outcomes seem to be uniform also at an international level, as shown by Bzowyckyj and Janke [5].

The objectives of education leading to the degrees of Bachelor's and Master's of Science (Pharmacy) are: (1) To produce experts for pharmaceutical work in all branches of healthcare and provide the knowledge and skills needed to maintain and improve their expertise; (2) To ensure pharmaceutical expertise, the degrees aim to provide students with the general knowledge and skills described below. Directive 2005/36/EC outlines the knowledge to be acquired through the education leading to the Master's of Science (Pharmacy) degree.

Table 1. Learning outcomes for the degrees of Bachelor's and Master's of Science (Pharmacy).

Bachelor's of Science (Pharmacy)	
Learning outcomes concerning knowledge of students who have completed the degree:	Learning outcomes concerning generic skills of students who have completed the degree:
Can apply basic knowledge of the natural sciences and biomedicine in pharmaceutical work	Have developed a professional identity and understand their expert role and duties in healthcare
Have a comprehensive command of pharmacotherapy, from the manufacture of medications to their safe and appropriate use	Are capable of critical thinking, that is, can assess information and apply the results of research in their work
Understand the field of pharmacy as a whole, including employment prospects as well as the role and significance of pharmacy in Finnish and other societies and healthcare systems	Have good problem-solving skills, can tolerate uncertainty, and can acquire information independently
Have the language and communication skills required for expert pharmaceutical work	Understand the necessity of lifelong learning, are motivated to enhance their expertise and can act in a self-directed, creative, ethical, and responsible manner in compliance with the principles of sustainable development
Understand the basic economic principles of business operations and the social functions of healthcare	Can communicate and interact both with customers and in multi-professional groups
Master's of Science (Pharmacy)	
Learning outcomes concerning knowledge	Learning outcomes concerning generic skills
Students who have completed the degree have expanded the knowledge and skills acquired through their Bachelor's of Science (Pharmacy) degree, in addition to which they:	
Profoundly understand the broad scope of the discipline of pharmacy and have a command of its key phenomena, theories, and concepts	Can work as experts, trainers, and developers in multiprofessional groups in both the pharmaceutical industry and the healthcare sector in Finland and abroad
Have a command of the basics of pharmaceutical development, understand the process of pharmaceutical development, and can apply their knowledge as experts in pharmaceutical development and pharmacotherapy	Have a command of key research methods as well as the research-based work method, can draw scientific conclusions and can produce scientific texts
Have acquired good theoretical competence and methodological knowledge in their specialist area	Have acquired the competences needed for research work in their specialist area as well as the competences for independent work in an international multi-professional research community
Can work in an expert environment in compliance with the principles of expert leadership and have the competence to develop in supervisory positions	Can think critically and analytically and apply research-based knowledge in their work, and have acquired good argumentation and problem-solving skills
Have a command of the basic concepts of business administration and understand the realities of business, particularly from the perspective of pharmaceutical medicine	Understand the potential provided by their expertise in various international environments

3.2. Curriculum Structures

In order to meet the defined learning outcomes and to foster the constructive alignment in teaching, the curriculum structure was modified first. For the Bachelor's program (the first three study years), a strand model was created by grouping the courses with similar contents to the same strand, to diminish the overlapping of the courses and to promote the smooth continuum of the studies (Figure 2). Coordinators for the four strands in the curriculum, the strand leaders, were nominated in 2014 to lead this process and to develop the constructive alignment and collaboration in the curriculum development and practices. To increase the professional identity of the pharmacy students, the amount of optional studies was increased in the new curriculum. In addition, the optional studies were grouped into three study paths, namely (1) community and hospital pharmacy; (2) industrial pharmacy and pharmaceutical authorities; and (3) research and scientific thinking.

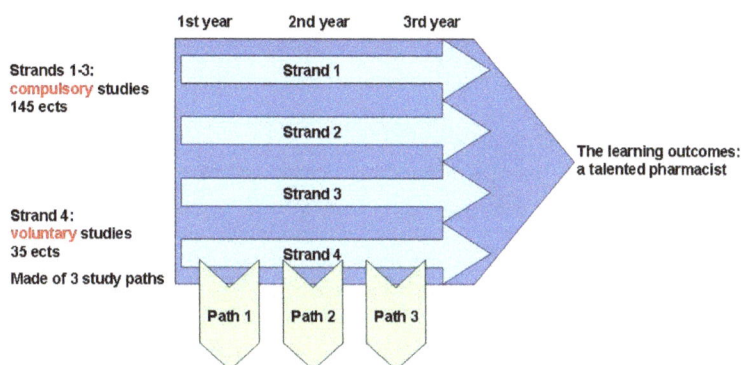

Figure 2. The strand model in Bachelor's program in the University of Helsinki.

During the Master's program (fourth and fifth study years) the first autumn includes compulsory studies incorporated to one large module, called "Drug Development and Use" (Figure 3). Parallel to this module, there are other compulsory modules including business, economics, analytics and statistics, and also preparation of a personal learning portfolio. The whole term is implemented in close collaboration of all the responsible teachers lead by a named coordinator. In the beginning of the spring term, the students select one specializing study line from seven different disciplines within the field of pharmacy. During these advanced major subject studies the students prepare their Master's Thesis. The program also contains advanced level optional studies.

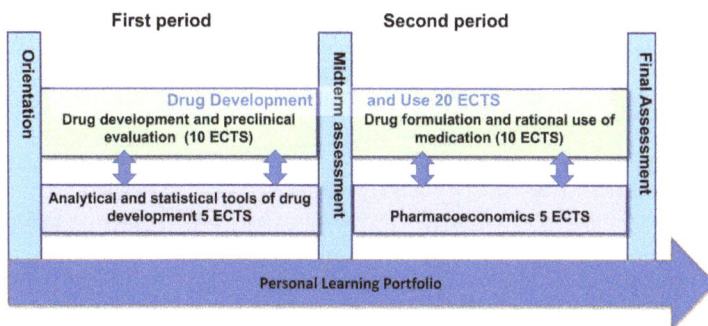

Figure 3. The compulsory studies during the fourth year of Master's Program in Pharmacy in the University of Helsinki.

As a result of the Big Wheel reform, steering groups with degree program directors were nominated for the Bachelor's and Master's programs in the end of the year 2016. These groups co-operate with each other and lead all the teaching and education development practices from now on, while different working groups, like strand leaders, fall within the guidance of these steering groups.

3.3. Projects Based on the Defined Learning Outcomes during the Pharmacy Education

A few projects extending over the whole curriculum were established to respond to the requested theoretical and generic learning outcomes, and further, to foster students' deep-level learning:

(1) teachers' workshops within and between the strands in Bachelor's program and during the first term of the Master's program; (2) student group work emphasizing the generic skills; (3) portfolio working; (4) progress testing; and (5) the proof demonstration of knowledge/skills.

3.3.1. Engagement of the Teachers to Constructive Alignment in Curriculum Design

In order to foster the co-operation in teaching and to develop the teaching and assessment methods, the new strand model and the modules in the programs were discussed and developed in workshops lead by the nominated strand leaders (see [14,16,17]). The new learning outcomes of the programs were implemented and defined also for the strands and individual courses. Several workshops within the strands and modules were carried out including discussions between the teachers about the learning outcomes, constructive alignment, teaching, and assessing methods which would foster students' deep level learning, challenge-level of the studies and the work-load of the learning tasks.

These workshops created an enthusiastic atmosphere between the teachers. Co-operation and alignment between courses were achieved and teaching and assessment methods were developed. The amount of the lectures was reduced, and new teaching methods like flipped classroom, different assignments, and projects, were introduced to the courses. Assessment methods were also diversified to include also self and peer evaluation, oral assessment, and evaluation of the project works. In addition, the timing of the teaching and assessments were coordinated (see [8]).

From now on, the nominated steering groups of the programs followed the work of the teachers in the strand groups as well as in the module groups and make sure that the teaching and evaluation of the programs were based on the learning outcomes and followed the principles of constructive alignment.

3.3.2. Fostering the Learning of Generic Skills

In order to help students to achieve the defined learning outcomes, to encourage their deep-level learning, and to achieve generic skills (Table 1), a systematic and explicit approach was integrated to the theoretical studies facilitating students' active learning process (see [8–10]).

In the very beginning of their studies, students are divided into small groups. Within these groups, they study together the whole academic year practicing generic skills and solving complicated theoretical problems related to theoretical courses. Four challenging theoretical courses throughout the first study year were selected for this purpose. Each course has a specific theme for the generic skills exercises like group forming, learning methods and scheduling, presentation of results of the assignments, and preparation for an examination. Instructions for the groups are given via the Moodle learning environment during the courses and the groups work independently on assignments without teachers. With proper instructions and well-thought exercises the students are able to work in groups without tutoring and solve the theoretical problems given in the courses.

Student groups produce materials and memorandums to the Moodle. In these memos, students reflect on their study process and present solutions for the theoretical assignments. The students' outputs are addressed during the lectures afterwards and the teachers also give feedback of the tasks collectively via the Moodle.

The group meetings succeeded well and the students felt that the groups are effective in helping to understand the theory and to learn generic skills. On the other hand, some students have had problems in understanding the significance of the group work and allocating time for the meetings. Teachers' experiences have been positive: students' study success and group working skills have been significantly improved compared to previous years, and less individual tutoring is needed. In the future, the group assignments will be developed further by selecting the most relevant and closely connected assignments to the theoretical courses. The solid basis for group working is established during the first study year. Different kinds of group assignments continue throughout the study program. In the second study year, learning of the generic skills is highlighted by different kinds of self-evaluations related to the theoretical courses.

3.3.3. The Learning Portfolio in the Study Programs

A portfolio is a tool to plan and document ones' education, work demonstrations and skills. A portfolio can include in-depth reflection of ones' development and transferable skills. In higher education, portfolios can be used as a tool to evaluate how well the theoretical and generic skills are achieved during the curriculum [18,19].

In order to visualize the learning and development of the students, a portfolio for the pharmacy programs was introduced (Table 2). In the portfolio, the student reflects on his/her learning with respect to the learning outcomes twice during the academic year. In addition, the student makes personal plans for studies, reflects on learning skills, completes the progress test (Section 3.3.4.) once a year, and summarizes the overall development during the studies via the demonstration of proof (Section 3.3.5). Also, the student reflects his/her knowledge and skills with regards to future employment. In the Master's program, the student also writes an application with a motivation letter for the main discipline for their advanced studies. All these assignments and instructions are given via Moodle.

Table 2. The contents of the student portfolio of the pharmacy programs.

Portfolio of the Pharmacy Programs
Reflection of learning in respect to the learning outcomes
Student's personal study plans
Reflection of the student's learning skills
Progress testing
Summarization of the development (years 1–3)
Demonstration of proof
Application for the main discipline with a motivation letter
Summarization of the development (years 4–5)

3.3.4. Progress Testing throughout the Curriculum

A progress test is a longitudinal educational assessment tool which gives feedback to both the student and the teacher about the development of knowledge during the learning process. The progress test is comprised of multiple choice questions, which assess the substance-specific knowledge, and is administered to all students at the same time at regular intervals throughout the program studies. The differences between students' knowledge level is shown in the test scores: the further a student has progressed in the curriculum, the higher the score. The results of the progress test provide a longitudinal, repeated assessment of the success on theoretical learning outcomes of the entire curriculum [20–22].

In the Faculty of Pharmacy, the strand leaders evaluate the results of the progress test. The idea is based on multidisciplinary questions, which measure a deeper understanding of substance concepts and foster the multidisciplinary nature of the questions. The progress test was launched in spring 2015 and it has now been implemented during the first three years of studies. The test acts as an evaluation tool for the degree program, and the students are actively using the progress test to evaluate their own development. The teachers have already began to see which areas of theoretical studies are well learned and which need brushing up. The degree program directors have gained evidence for the development and improvement of the curriculum. Thus, the progress test works nicely in two ways, reciprocally, to aid both the students and teachers alike. Most importantly, by using the progress test, the degree program directors and the steering groups are able to monitor how well theoretical learning outcomes have been reached during the studies. Preliminary findings suggest that the student learning curve is improving steadily as the studies progress, and it seems that the predetermined learning outcomes can indeed be reached by the end of the studies.

3.3.5. The Demonstration of Proof

During the reform process, a practical test called the 'demonstration of proof' was created to evaluate both the theoretical and generic skills developed throughout the curriculum, and will be launched for the very first time in spring 2017. The practical test is a two-phase two-day event based on group work. The first phase will include group discussions about the development and strengths of students during their studies and with regards to their employment in the future. In the second phase, the students are given an inspirational stimulus describing a real-life challenge in the field of pharmacy. The students need to create a solution to the challenge, which could be an innovation, a product, a practice, or a procedure, which could be implemented further. The students need to use the theoretical knowledge and generic skills they have learned during their studies and work as a team, just like in real working life. The students will present their solutions to a panel, which consists of teachers and stakeholders. The panel evaluates the students' presentations and rewards the most innovative and creative solutions.

The aim of this practical is to summarize the theoretical and generic learning outcomes of the study program. Never before have the learning outcomes been assessed at the end of the studies as a whole. The constructive alignment of the teaching and assessment methods should be implemented not only at the course level, but also in the program level. A final book exam, or even a practical exam, which only measures learning-by-heart type learning, does not answer properly to the question of how learning outcomes have been reached. It is more likely that this type of group activity will demonstrate better the constructive alignment and the achievement of the learning outcomes. The intention is to develop a similar kind of practice for the Master's program as well. [3,8,13,23].

4. Conclusions

During the reform process, it became clear that it is absolutely necessary to involve all the stakeholders including teachers and students when reforming the curriculum. Although the reform process was demanding and time-consuming, it was inspiring at the same time. Even though the process was unforeseeable, the teams could hold the processes together by carefully managing, planning, and changing them in the case of altering circumstances.

The reform process was able to produce the intended learning outcomes. For the first time in Helsinki, the learning outcomes for the programs in pharmacy included also the generic skills, in addition to the theoretical skills. The learning outcomes enable the curriculum to be built based on constructive alignment and to create the knowledge and skills needed in working life. Increased co-operation with the stakeholders will aid in reaching the intended learning outcomes.

In the Faculty of Pharmacy, many processes—such as workshops for teachers, organized group work for students, learning portfolios, progress tests, and demonstration of proof—were developed in order to foster student's deep-level learning, to visualize the development of the students, to evaluate and reach the learning outcomes, to ensure the implementation of the constructive alignment and high quality of the study programs. In order to secure the quality of the programs and to create a sense of community and co-operation between the teachers, it is important to nominate committed responsible persons for the sub-structures of the curriculum. In the Faculty of Pharmacy, the nominated program directors with steering groups and strand leaders follow up and make sure that the programs fulfill the criteria of high quality education.

The University of Helsinki has participated and kept a keen eye on European level educational development, especially the Pharmine and PHAR-QA projects. Health and patient care orientations and development of generic skills, in addition to subject specific knowledge of drugs, are megatrends that request active follow-up, pedagogic capacity, and active measures to keep pharmacy education as one of the front-runners in University education.

Author Contributions: Nina Katajavuori made a first version of the manuscript which was written together with Outi Salminen and Katariina Vuorensola. Jouni Hirvonen commented and finalized the manuscript and Helena Huhtala and Pia Vuorela commented the manuscript.

Conflicts of Interest: The authors declare no conflict of interest.

References

1. International Pharmaceutical Federation. Fip Statement of Policy on Good Pharmacy Education Practice. 2000. Available online: http://www.fip.org/www/uploads/database_file.php?id=188&table_id= (accessed on 25 March 2017).
2. Fallows, S.; Steven, C. Building employability skills into the higher education curriculum: A university-wide initiative. *Educ. Train.* **2000**, *42*, 75–83. [CrossRef]
3. Biggs, J.; Tang, C. *Teaching for Quality Learning at University: What the Student Does*, 2nd ed.; Society for Research into Higher Education & Open University Press: Buckingham, UK, 2003.
4. Tynjälä, P.; Slotte, V.; Nieminen, J.; Lonka, K.; Olkinuora, E. From University to working life: Graduates' workplace skills in practice. In *Higher Education and Working life—Collaborations, Confrontations and Challenges*; Tynjälä, P., Välimaa, J., Boulton-Lewis, G., Eds.; Elsevier: Amsterdam, The Netherlands, 2006; pp. 77–88.
5. Bzowyckyj, A.S.; Janke, K.K. A Consensus Definition and Core Competencies for Being an Advocate for Pharmacy. *Am. J. Pharm. Educ.* **2013**, *77*, 24. [CrossRef] [PubMed]
6. Weinert, F.E. Concept of Competence: A Conceptual clarification. In *Defining and Selecting Key Competencies*; Rychen, D.S., Sagalnik, L.H., Eds.; Hogrefe & Huber: Seattle, WA, USA, 2001.
7. Frank, J.R.; Snell, L.S.; Cate, O.T.; Holmboe, E.S.; Carraccio, C.; Swing, S.R.; Harris, P.; Glasgow, N.J.; Campbell, C.; Dath, D.; et al. Competency-based medical education: Theory to practice. *Med. Teach.* **2010**, *32*, 638–645. [CrossRef] [PubMed]
8. Biggs, J.; Tang, C. *Teaching for Quality Learning at University*, 4th ed.; Society for Research into Higher Education & Open University Press: Buckingham, UK, 2011.
9. Jones, A. Generic attributes as espoused theory: The importance of context. *High. Educ.* **2009**, *58*, 175–191.
10. Badcock, P.B.T.; Philippa, E.P.; Harris, K.-L. Developing generic skills through university study: A study of arts, science and engineering in Australia. *High. Educ.* **2010**, *60*, 441–458. [CrossRef]
11. Tuxworth, E. Competence based education and training: Backgroung and origins. In *Competence Based Education and Training*; Burke, J.W., Ed.; Falmer Press: Sussex, UK, 1989.
12. Kemper, D. Nurturing generic capabilities through a teaching and learning environment which provides practise in their use. *High. Educ.* **2009**, *57*, 37–55. [CrossRef]
13. Biggs, J. Enhancing teaching through constructive alignment. *High. Educ.* **1996**, *32*, 1–18. [CrossRef]
14. Shulman, L. Teaching as community property. *Change* **1993**, *25*, 6–7. [CrossRef]
15. Kahn, P.; Goodhew, P.; Murphy, M.; Walsh, L. The Scholarship of Teaching and Learning as collaborative working: A case study in shared practice and collective purpose. *High. Educ. Res. Dev.* **2013**, *32*, 901–914. [CrossRef]
16. Davis, B. A conceptual model to Support Curriculum Review, Revision, and Design in an Associate Degree Nursing Program. *Nurs. Educ. Perspect. (Natl. Leag. Nurs.)* **2011**, *32*, 389–394. [CrossRef]
17. Lakkala, M.; Toom, A.; Ilomäki, L.; Muukkonen, H. Re-designing university courses to support collaborative knowledge creation practices. *Australas. J. Educ. Tech.* **2015**, *31*, 521–536. [CrossRef]
18. Tillema, H.H. Portfolios as Developmental Assessment Tools. *Int. J. Train. Dev.* **2001**, *5*, 126–135. [CrossRef]
19. Gadbury-Amyot, C.C.; Bray, K.K.; Austin, K.J. Fifteen years of portfolio assessment of dental hygiene student competency: Lessons learned. *J. Dent. Hyg.* **2014**, *88*, 267–274. [PubMed]
20. Van Diest, R.; Dalen, J.V.; Bak, M.; Schruers, K.; Vleuten, C.V.D.; Muijtjens, A.; Scherpbier, A. Growth of knowledge in psychiatry and behavioural sciences in a problem-based learning curriculum. *Med. Educ.* **2004**, *38*, 1295–1301. [CrossRef] [PubMed]
21. Verhoeven, B.H.; Snellen-Balendong, H.A.; Hay, I.T.; Boon, J.M.; van der Linde, M.J.; Blitz-Lindeque, J.J.; Hoogenboom, R.J.I.; Verwijnen, G.M.; Wijnen, W.H.F.W.; Scherpbier, A.J.J.A.; et al. The versatility of progress testing assessed in an international context: A start for benchmarking global standardization? *Med. Teach.* **2005**, *27*, 514–520. [CrossRef] [PubMed]
22. Freeman, A.; van der Vleuten, C.; Nouns, Z.; Ricketts, C. Progress testing internationally. *Med. Teach.* **2010**, *32*, 451–455. [CrossRef] [PubMed]
23. Biggs, J. What the student does: Teaching for enhanced learning. *High. Educ. Res. Dev.* **1999**, *18*, 57–75. [CrossRef]

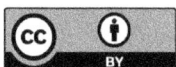

![pharmacy logo] *pharmacy*

MDPI

Article

The Implementation of Pharmacy Competence Teaching in Estonia

Daisy Volmer [1,*], **Kristiina Sepp** [2], **Peep Veski** [1,†] **and Ain Raal** [1]

[1]   Institute of Pharmacy, University of Tartu, Nooruse 1, 50411 Tartu, Estonia; ain.raal@ut.ee (A.R.)
[2]   Estonian Pharmacies Association; Vae 16, Laagri, 76401 Harju County, Estonia; kristiina.sepp@apotheka.ee
*   Correspondence: daisy.volmer@ut.ee; Tel.: +372-7-375-298
†   Greatly involved in curriculum development

Academic Editor: Jeffrey Atkinson
Received: 22 January 2017; Accepted: 27 March 2017; Published: 31 March 2017

Abstract: Background: The PHAR-QA, "Quality Assurance in European Pharmacy Education and Training", project has produced the European Pharmacy Competence Framework (EPCF). The aim of this study was to evaluate the existing pharmacy programme at the University of Tartu, using the EPCF. **Methods:** A qualitative assessment of the pharmacy programme by a convenience sample ($n = 14$) representing different pharmacy stakeholders in Estonia. EPCF competency levels were determined by using a five-point scale tool adopted from the Dutch competency standards framework. Mean scores of competency levels given by academia and other pharmacy stakeholders were compared. **Results:** Medical and social sciences, pharmaceutical technology, and pharmacy internship were more frequent subject areas contributing to EPCF competencies. In almost all domains, the competency level was seen higher by academia than by other pharmacy stakeholders. Despite on-board theoretical knowledge, the competency level at graduation could be insufficient for independent professional practice. Other pharmacy stakeholders would improve practical implementation of theoretical knowledge, especially to increase patient care competencies. **Conclusions:** The EPCF was utilized to evaluate professional competencies of entry-level pharmacists who have completed a traditional pharmacy curriculum. More efficient training methods and involvement of practicing specialists were suggested to reduce the gaps of the existing pharmacy programme. Applicability of competence teaching in Estonia requires more research and collaborative communication within the pharmacy sector.

Keywords: competence; competency; pharmacy education; Estonia

---

1. Introduction

1.1. Pharmacy Education and Training in Estonia

The Faculty of Medicine at the University of Tartu (UT), Estonia, provides higher education and several PhD programmes in medicine, dentistry, pharmacy, sport sciences, and physiotherapy [1]. Pharmacists (*proviisor* in Estonian) study at the UT for five years and graduate with a Masters of Pharmacy (MSc Pharm) (Figure 1). Pharmacists can be owners and managers of community pharmacies, work as responsible pharmacists in the community and hospital pharmacies, or other pharmacy fields (e.g., wholesale companies or in the pharmaceutical industry). Effective as of 2020, the ownership of community pharmacies will be limited to the pharmacy profession (more than 50 per cent of the shares have to belong to pharmacists). Currently, the majority of community pharmacies have joined different pharmacy chains and mainly traditional services (e.g., dispensing and counselling of the use of prescription and non-prescription medicines) have been provided. In addition, different extended services (e.g., diagnostic clinical tests) have developed [2]. Assistant pharmacists (*farmatseut* in Estonian) study at Tallinn Healthcare College for three years and are mainly employed in community pharmacies after graduation [3]. Specialists with a diploma of assistant pharmacist who want to continue their education and become pharmacists have to pass the full five-year programme at UT. All practicing pharmacists and assistant pharmacists have to be registered at the corresponding professional register and have to participate in the continuing professional development (CPD) courses for at least 40 h over two years [4] (Figure 1).

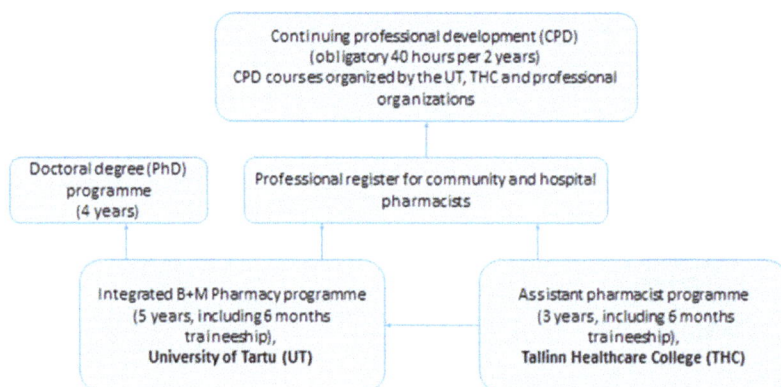

Figure 1. The pharmacy education and continuing professional development scheme in Estonia.

The pharmacy programme at UT is designed as medical subject-based and pharmaceutical product-oriented, following the sectorial profession model and the EU directives [5,6]. The curriculum is organized as a course based on five years of integrated bachelor and master training (300 ECTS). The existing pharmacy programme is the basis for recognition of professional qualification. Currently the pharmacy curriculum is available only in Estonian and does not offer specialization. However, international students could participate in research work or take single courses based on individual learning and examination [7].

The pharmacy programme is constantly reviewed and modified. The proportion of in-class lectures has decreased, while independent work has increased; problem-based and research-based training have been introduced in some subjects. The proportion of chemistry-based subjects has decreased and the amount of pharmaceutical technology and medical subjects has increased. A large proportion of medical subjects in the pharmacy programme was intended to prepare future pharmacists for more efficient collaboration in health care teams. During the last ten years, interdisciplinary subjects such as pharmacoeconomics and pharmacoepidemiology, biotechnology, genetics, and bioethics have been integrated into the programme. The patient care concept has been introduced by subjects such as primary care medicine, laboratory medicine, clinical microbiology, clinical pharmacology, and clinical pharmacy (the last subject was added in 2017) (see Appendix A). A comparison of the pharmacy programme of the UT with respective pharmacy curricula in the EU is presented in Table 1 [8].

Table 1. Comparison of seven subject areas in pharmacy programmes in EU and UT, Estonia.

Subject Area	Proportion of Subject Areas in Pharmacy Programmes EU Main %	Proportion of Subject Areas in the Pharmacy Programme (UT), Estonia %
Chemical sciences	26	21
Physics, mathematics	6	4
Biological sciences	11	2
Pharmaceutical technology	16	21
Medical sciences	28	39
Law and social sciences	7	10
Generic subjects, traineeship	6	3

In the Pharmacy programme, four subject groups—drug analysis (chemistry subjects and pharmacognosy), pharmaceutical technology, medical, and social sciences—have been identified (Table 2). Continuity of the subject areas is organized by the system of pre-subjects: subjects placed in the earlier years of training are pre-requisite subjects for the following, and more specialized, subjects (see Appendix A).

Table 2. Distribution of subject groups within first four study years in the pharmacy programme (UT).

Study Year	Drug Analysis	Pharmaceutical Technology	Medical Sciences and Patient Care Subjects	Social Sciences
First	Inorganic and analytical chemistry	-	Anatomy, physiology, medical microbiology	Latin, pharmaceutical terminology, history of pharmacy
Second	Analytical, bioorganic and pharmaceutical chemistry	Pharmaceutical excipients	Physiology, pathophysiology, clinical microbiology, medical biochemistry, genetics, primary care medicine	Bioethics
Third	Pharmacognosy, pharmaceutical chemistry	Pharmaceutical technology, biotechnology	Laboratory medicine, pharmacology	-
Fourth	Metabolism of active substances	Physical pharmacy, biopharmacy	Immunology, pharmacotherapy, first aid, drug toxicology, clinical pharmacology, clinical pharmacy,	Pharmaco- epidemiology and pharmaco-economics,social pharmacy, and drug safety

1.2. How to Achieve Competency Based Pharmacy Education in Estonia?

Current pharmacy programme at the UT is compiled using a traditional subject and course-based system. Identification and description of the "flow chart" of subject areas in the pharmacy programme could be seen as a start to describe the curriculum by competencies. The next possible step could be the connection of subject areas with particular entry-level pharmacist professional competencies in the future.

Another possibility to collect valuable information for development of pharmacy training could be to use professional guidelines, e.g., "Community pharmacy service quality guidelines" [9] and "Estonian hospital pharmacy good practices" [10] that were developed and implemented in 2012 and 2015, respectively. Both guidelines shape the expected quality of pharmacy practice in community and hospital setting in Estonia. Community pharmacy guidelines list the indicators that every community pharmacy could use for self-assessment of its pharmacy operation and service provisions. Guideline based self-assessment reports have showed community pharmacists to have higher confidence about providing traditional rather than extended services. Patient-centred counselling of medicines and the provision of extended services are impeded by the shortage of professional personnel, the lack of private consultation possibilities at pharmacies, lack of motivation towards treatment, and use of medicines among patients, as well as by the insufficient professional competency of community pharmacists [2].

Changes within pharmacy profession competencies include moving from product- to patient-oriented knowledge and skills. More attention has to be paid to patient-centred pharmaceutical care services. There are several existing frameworks for evaluating changes in the performance and competence of practicing pharmacists [11–16]. For entry-level pharmacists, competency guidelines based on curriculum outcomes have been developed in Canada, Australia, and the UK [17–19]. The European Pharmacy Competence Framework (EPCF) has been produced within the project PHAR-QA, "Quality Assurance in European Pharmacy Education and Training", as a new assessment tool for competency-based pharmacy training in Europe [20].

The aim of this study was to evaluate the existing pharmacy programme at the UT by using the EPCF:

- to construct a curriculum mapping matrix;
- to assess the pharmacy curriculum outcome based competency level, and
- to identify the pharmacy curriculum gaps and evaluate the expediency of the EPCF as a curriculum mapping tool.

2. Materials and Methods

2.1. PHAR-QA Framework

The EPCF was produced by EU project PHAR-QA, "Quality Assurance in European Pharmacy Education and Training". Developed tool includes personal and patient care competences presented in 11 domains and 50 particularly defined competences (Appendix B). The tool has been validated in a two-round Delphi survey by more than 2000 representatives of different pharmacy stakeholders in Europe [21,22]. For the implementation of the EPCF, it was important to learn its usability as a guideline for evaluation and development of pharmacy curricula in the EU. UT, Institute of Pharmacy, acted as a partner in the PHAR-QA project, and volunteered to pilot the tool for the evaluation of the pharmacy programme.

2.2. Study Design and Sample

The initial study design was developed and proposed by Prof. Andries Koster, University of Utrecht, Utrecht, Netherlands [23]. Among pharmacy schools piloting the EPCF, the following study structure was agreed upon:

- intended (existing) curriculum mapping: matrix construction of 50 EPCF competences and curriculum elements;
- evaluation of expected competency level at the graduation of first-degree curriculum (MSc degree); and
- identification of curriculum gaps.

A qualitative assessment of the pharmacy programme was performed and a convenience sample of different pharmacy stakeholders was involved: academia (teaching staff at the Institute of Pharmacy), wholesale and retail sale of medicines, hospital pharmacy, representatives of pharmaceutical industry, and other fields (e.g., State Agency of Medicines).

Instead of studying pharmacy students' perception about the competency-based curriculum, the decision was to involve recently graduated pharmacists who could analyse the pharmacy programme from the point of view of both students and pharmacists. Fourteen evaluators (seven from academia and seven from other pharmacy fields) participated in the assessment. Six of the respondents had graduated recently (1–5 years ago) and eight were experienced specialists.

2.3. Data Analysis

As some of the EPCF competences were supported by more than one pharmacy programme subject, evaluators decided to use different types of curriculum elements (subjects, subject areas, and full programme) in the mapping exercise. The subject area was defined by using previously-determined subject groups (Table 2). In the evaluation, all pharmacy programme subjects (obligatory and elective) were used. Detailed description of the pharmacy programme at UT is presented in Appendix A.

Based on the outcomes of curriculum elements and evaluators' own practical experience, the competency levels were identified according to the personal and patient care competences listed in EPCF. A five-point scale tool, adopted from the Dutch competency standards framework [23] and based on the increase of professional independence, was used as follows:

- 1: Theoretical education; LEVEL OF INDEPENDENCE 1;
- 2: Theoretical education and practical skills; LEVEL OF INDEPENDENCE 2;
- 3: Ability to use theoretical knowledge and practical skills in learning situations; LEVEL OF INDEPENDENCE 3;
- 4: Ability to use theoretical knowledge and practical skills in authentic learning situations (classroom and during pharmacy internship); LEVEL OF INDEPENDENCE 4;
- 5: Ability to use theoretical knowledge and practical skills in practice; LEVEL OF INDEPENDENCE.

The required competency level for recent pharmacy programme graduates at UT could start with a professional independence level 3 and higher. The mean values for 11 competence domains based on the described five-point scale assessment tool were calculated and the results of academia and other pharmacy stakeholders were compared.

In this article the term "competence" is used to describe knowledge and skills—standards—needed to reach professional performance. The term "competency" describes behaviour and commitment in achieving competences.

3. Results

3.1. Construction of Curriculum Mapping Matrix

Table 3 shows developed matrix based on the 11 competence domains of the EPCF and the pharmacy programme elements. EPCF personal competences were mostly covered by the full programme with emphasis on some subject areas. The EPCF patient care competences were supported by specific subject areas or specific subjects, and the number of subjects covering these competences increased with study years. The existing pharmacy programme included subjects and subject areas in logical order and, thus, supported the generation of professional competency. More frequent subject areas for reaching the 50 EPCF competences were medical and social sciences, pharmaceutical technology, and pharmacy internship. Medical and social sciences both contributed to 40% and pharmacy internship to 30% of the listed competences. Elective subjects covered personal as well as patient care competences. In some cases, the competence was supported mostly by the elective courses, e.g., the domain "patient education".

Not all of the EPCF competences were covered with the pharmacy programme subjects. For example: the business and entrepreneurship competences ("ability to identify the need for new services" and "ability to understand a business environment and develop entrepreneurship") have not been covered by any of the curriculum subjects. The competences about drug registration and marketing; supply chain of medicines, and public health issues have been very briefly taught in different obligatory and elective subjects.

Table 3. EPCF and the pharmacy programme (UT) based curriculum mapping matrix and mean values of competency levels assessed by representatives of academia and other pharmacy stakeholders.

Competence Domains	Specific Subjects	Subject Area/-s	Full Programme	Mean Competency Level *, Academia	Mean Competency Level *, Other Pharmacy Stakeholders
Personal competences					
1. Learning and knowledge	NA **	Medical and social sciences, pharmacy internship	Yes	4.0	3.4
2. Values	NA	Social sciences, pharmacy internship	Yes	4.4	3.7
3. Communication and organizational skills	NA	Social sciences, pharmacy internship	Yes	3.8	3.1
4. Research and industrial pharmacy	Yes	Pharmaceutical technology, drug analysis	Yes, only one competence	4.0	2.5
Personal competence domains 1–4 mean value				**4.1**	**3.2**
Patient care competences					
5. Patient consultation and assessment	Yes	Medical sciences	NA	3.3	3.2
6. Need for drug treatment	Yes	Medical sciences	NA	3.0	3.0
7. Drug interactions	Yes	Medical sciences, pharmaceutical technology	NA	3.0	3.2
8. Drug dose and formulation	Yes	Pharmaceutical technology, medical sciences	NA	4.2	3.0
9. Patient education	Yes	No	NA	4.0	3.7
10. Provision of information and service	Yes	Medical and social sciences, pharmaceutical technology, pharmacy internship	NA	4.7	3.5
11. Monitoring of drug therapy	Yes	Medical and social sciences, pharmaceutical technology, pharmacy internship	NA	3.2	2.4
Patient care competence domains 5–11 mean value				**3.6**	**3.1**

* Five-point competency level evaluation scale: 1-theoretical education and 5-ability to use independently theoretical knowledge and practical skills in practice; ** NA—not applicable.

117

3.2. Competencies of Entry-Level Pharmacists

In both academia and other pharmacy stakeholders' groups the level of personal competencies was assessed higher than patient care competencies (Table 3). In almost all domains, the competency level was perceived to be at a higher level by academia than the pharmacy sector representatives. The latter evaluated personal and patient care competency level as three on the five-point scale. The academia group rated personal competency level higher (four on a five-point scale), but agreed with the pharmacy sector group on patient care competency level. The two groups disagreed the most on the level of personal competencies in the domain "research and industrial pharmacy". Considerable variations were identified in patient care competency levels in two domains: "drug dose and formulation" and "provision of information and service".

3.3. Curriculum Gaps

Both groups of evaluators described more and less positive aspects of the pharmacy programme. An expansive education was expected to support critical thinking and logical problem solving, large proportion of medical subjects, and the involvement of practicing specialists from different pharmacy fields were emphasized as good basis for contemporary higher education.

Representatives of different pharmacy sectors addressed several issues in the pharmacy programme organization and training methods:

- increase collaboration between different healthcare professions; more integrated training and common courses with medical students;
- support more patient care competencies linking the pharmacy programme with practice on different fields of pharmacy starting already from the first years of studies;
- support the reflection and practical implementation of theoretical knowledge, more broad use of problem-based learning in different subjects;
- introduce business and entrepreneurship subjects to the pharmacy programme as from 2020, pharmacy ownership will be limited only by pharmacy profession in Estonia;
- develop more detailed requirements for pharmacy students and for internship supervisors at community and hospital pharmacies as pharmacy internship plays very important role in implementing of professional competencies.

3.4. Usability of EPCF in Curriculum Mapping and Competency Level Evaluation

The EPCF was utilized to identify competencies that have not been covered by the existing pharmacy programme or competencies that were not sufficiently supported by existing subjects. As the EPCF has been designed with a focus on professional competencies required in community pharmacy, this could, to some extent, impede using this type of tool for evaluation of the curriculum without specialization. This kind of training focuses on providing as broad professional knowledge as possible and does not concentrate in detail only on patient care competencies. For competency level evaluation, a proposal was made to use the five-step Dutch competency standards framework because Miller's 'pyramid' (knows, knows how, shows how, and does) does not provide a detailed description of professional knowledge and independence of pharmacists on different competency levels. To address more country-specific needs, other evaluation methods could be considered or developed in future.

4. Discussion

This was the first time the use a competency-based model has been applied for the evaluation of the pharmacy programme at the UT. The assessment provided important information and it is in line with the recommendations presented by an international accreditation team of the Medicine Study Programme Group at UT in 2014 [24]. Both evaluations stressed the need for integrated and novel training methods, for self-reflection and analysis of acquired knowledge by students and for more frequent collaboration between practicing specialists so theoretical knowledge could be implemented into practice better.

Gradual implementation of medical subjects to the pharmacy programme was planned to increase professional competency of pharmacists as healthcare professionals. Based on the EPCF evaluation, the medical subjects of the existing pharmacy programme might not provide sufficient support to patient care competencies in terms of practical usability. However, the description of professional competencies for pharmacists and assistant pharmacists had been missing for the past two decades in Estonia and this situation was not conductive to providing practice-linked training. In November 2016, the occupational qualification standards for pharmacists and assistant pharmacists were approved in Estonia [25]. The standards enable clear identification of professional roles within the pharmacy profession and provide detailed descriptions of required competencies. This kind of supporting information will be vital for the advancement of pharmacy education in Estonia in future.

Representatives of the academia and other pharmacy stakeholders gave different scores to EPCF personal and patient care competencies level. Level of personal competencies was evaluated with a higher score than level of patient care competencies. As many of personal competences were seen as covered by the full pharmacy programme, the level of evaluated competencies could be more speculative than in the case of patient care competences where specific subjects were listed to support the particular competence.

Although the common agreement was to analyse the existing pharmacy programme, the competency evaluation could be conducted on various levels: for academia as knowledge-delivered level and for other pharmacy stakeholders as mix of perceived (viewpoint of students) and realized (viewpoint of practicing specialists and employers) levels. For academia, the evaluation was based on assumptions about the use of theoretical knowledge in practice. Representatives of other pharmacy sectors were expecting not only theoretically competent specialists, but somebody who could perform and fluently use acquired professional knowledge in their specific field of pharmacy. The delivery of diverse educational content might be the reason for surprisingly large score variations given by academia and other pharmacy stakeholders to patient care competencies: "drug dose and formulation" and "provision of information and service". Both domains describe core competencies of the pharmacy profession and have to be covered by any type of pharmacy curriculum. However, training methods play an important role in the use of acquired knowledge. Case- and problem-based learning could assure more practical use of theoretical knowledge and help future specialists to settle into working life more easily. Pharmacists planning to work in particular areas could have the possibility of constructing a description or list of competencies that are of importance and could assist in their professional performance. This type of differential approach is described in the National Competency Standards Framework for Pharmacists in Australia and would help to elucidate what competencies have to be developed more at CPD courses [19].

The development and implementation of a competency based pharmacy curriculum is a long process and requires common understanding of the higher education institution, other partners in the pharmacy sector and governmental institutions about the demand for considerable change in pharmacy education.

The UT has recently paid a lot of attention to the improvement of teaching and learning quality and published principles of Good Practice of Learning and Good Practice of Teaching, which is a part of the university's good practices. The new practice stimulates students and university staff members to be motivated to teach and learn. In addition, students are encouraged to self-reflect and analyse their studies, which is very important feedback in outcome-oriented professional education [26,27]. Good Practice of Teaching encourages development of teaching communities and emphasises the following principles: excellent teaching is learning centred, based on a scientific way of thinking and cooperation, supports creativity and entrepreneurship, leads to self-analysis, and supports individual development and links learning to real life [27].

In addition to the redesigning of the teaching and learning practices, it is necessary to assure conditions for the provision of competency based clinical practice. The development of professional competency is a continuous process involving both under- and post-graduate education.

Limitations

For all evaluators, curriculum development was not their field of expertise. In the future, it would be necessary to consult with curriculum development specialists and education scientists at the UT about curriculum organization and novel training methods. Additionally, more pharmacy stakeholders have to be involved in discussions and the decision-making process in order to identify the needs for pharmacy competence teaching in Estonia.

5. Conclusions

The EPCF-based mapping exercise of the pharmacy programme at UT provided useful information regarding professional competencies of entry-level pharmacists who have completed traditional pharmacy curriculum. Most of the EPCF competence domains were covered by subjects, subject areas, or the full pharmacy programme. However, to assure independent and responsible patient-centred professional practice, personal and patient care competency levels at graduation could be higher. Representatives of academia and other pharmacy stakeholders concluded that the existing pharmacy programme is designed to provide broad theoretical knowledge, but more efficient training methods should be implemented and practicing specialists from different fields of pharmacy should participate in the teaching process to link theory with practice more efficiently.

Additional research and continuous collaboration within the pharmacy sector is important in order to understand what would the most applicable way to move towards competency-based pharmacy training in Estonia.

Acknowledgments: The authors would like to thank representatives of the UT: Karin Kogermann, Urve Paaver, Ivo Laidmäe, Andres Lust, and Janne Sepp, and other pharmacy stakeholders, Timo Danilov, Kertu Margus, Marko Tähnas, Liisa-Kai Pedosk, Anne-Greete Raadom, and Marika Saar for their contribution to the curriculum mapping exercise.

Author Contributions: K.S. and D.V. performed the experiments; D.V. analysed the data and wrote the initial version of the paper. K.S. and A.R. provided constructive criticism of the manuscript.

Conflicts of Interest: The authors declare no conflict of interest.

Appendix A

Table A1. Content of the curriculum Pharmacy for entrants at the University of Tartu, Estonia, of 2016/2017.

Pharmacy (300 ECTS)			
1. Compulsory subjects (224 ECTS)			
1.1 First course compulsory subjects (51 ECTS)			
ARFA.02.099	Analytical Chemistry	12	ECTS
ARAN.01.034	Anatomy	5	ECTS
ARFS.01.023	Biophysics	4	ECTS
LOKT.00.004	General and Inorganic Chemistry	6	ECTS
ARFS.01.063	Human Physiology	10	ECTS
ARFA.01.071	Introduction and History of Pharmacy	3	ECTS
FLKE.05.009	Latin in Pharmacy	3	ECTS
ARMB.00.001	Medical Microbiology	6	ECTS
ARFA.02.098	Pharmaceutical Terminology	3	ECTS
ARFA.01.072	Pharmacognosy I	3	ECTS
MTMS.01.085	Statistical Analysis	4	ECTS

Table A1. *Cont.*

Pharmacy (300 ECTS)			
1.2 Second course compulsory subjects (52 ECTS)			
ARFA.02.099	Analytical Chemistry	12	ECTS
ARFA.02.108	Bioethics	4	ECTS
ARBK.01.042	Bioorganic Chemistry	5	ECTS
ARMB.01.053	Clinical Microbiology	2	ECTS
ARMP.01.030	Genetics	3	ECTS
ARFS.01.063	Human Physiology	10	ECTS
ARBK.01.043	Medical Biochemistry	5	ECTS
ARMP.03.031	Pathophysiology	6	ECTS
ARFA.02.109	Pharmaceutical Chemistry I	9	ECTS
ARFA.02.103	Pharmaceutical Excipients	5	ECTS
ARPO.00.020	Primary Care Medicine	5	ECTS
1.3 Third course compulsory subjects (52 ECTS)			
ARMP.03.035	Biotechnology	3	ECTS
ARSK.03.017	Introduction to the Laboratory Medicine	2	ECTS
ARFA.02.112	Pharmaceutical Chemistry II	8	ECTS
ARFA.02.113	Pharmaceutical Technology	22	ECTS
ARFA.01.105	Pharmacognosy II	7	ECTS
ARFA.01.077	Pharmacognosy III	4	ECTS
ARFR.02.051	Pharmacology	11	ECTS
1.4 Fourth course compulsory subjects (51 ECTS)			
ARFA.02.144	Biopharmaceutics	5	ECTS
ARFR.03.018	Clinical Pharmacology	2	ECTS
ARFA.01.104	Clinical Pharmacy	3	ECTS
ARFR.02.034	Drug Toxicology	3	ECTS
ARKI.01.004	First Aid	3	ECTS
ARMP.02.016	Immunology	2	ECTS
ARFA.02.123	Metabolism of Active Substances	3	ECTS
ARFA.02.113	Pharmaceutical Technology	22	ECTS
ARFA.01.059	Pharmacoepidemiology and Pharmacoeconomics	3	ECTS
ARFR.02.052	Pharmacotherapy	5	ECTS
ARFA.02.122	Physical Pharmacy	6	ECTS
ARFA.01.082	Social Pharmacy and Drug Safety	11	ECTS
1.5 Fifth course (18 ECTS)			
ARFA.02.040	Designing of Research Work	1	ECTS
ARFA.02.044	Pharmaceutical Commodities	4	ECTS
ARFA.00.057	Research Work	6	ECTS
or ARFS.01.076	Diploma Work	6	ECTS
or ARBK.01.048	Research Work	6	ECTS
or ARMB.01.059	Diploma Work	6	ECTS
or ARFR.02.061	Diploma Work	6	ECTS
or ARAN.00.040	Research Project	6	ECTS
seminar of research (7 ECTS) or			
ARFA.02.117	Research Seminar on Pharmaceutical Chemistry	7	ECTS
ARFA.02.116	Research Seminar on Pharmaceutical Technology	7	ECTS
ARFA.01.078	Research Seminar on Pharmacognosy	7	ECTS
ARFA.01.080	Research Seminar on Social Pharmacy	7	ECTS
ARFA.01.096	Research Seminars on Clinical Pharmacy	7	ECTS
ARFA.02.118	Research Seminars on History of Pharmacy	7	ECTS
ARFS.01.075	Research Workshop of Physiology	7	ECTS
ARAN.02.027	Seminar on Histology	7	ECTS
ARBK.01.047	Seminars of Research in Medical Biochemistry	7	ECTS
ARMB.01.060	Seminars of Research in Medical Microbiology	7	ECTS
ARFR.02.060	Seminars of Research in Pharmacology	7	ECTS

Table A1. *Cont.*

Pharmacy (300 ECTS)			
2. *Elective courses (22 ECTS)*			
2.1 First course elective subjects (6 ECTS)			
FLKE.03.151	Estonian for Students of Medicine, on the Basis of Russian, Level B1 >B2	3	ECTS
ARFA.02.080	Exercises and Problems in Pharmaceutical Analysis	1	ECTS
ARLA.01.034	Foetal and Neonatal Physiology and Behaviour, Breastfeeding	2	ECTS
ARSK.00.009	Gerontology. Introduction (web-based)	3	ECTS
FLFI.00.002	Introduction to Philosophy	2	ECTS
ARFA.01.106	Pharmacist in pharmacy system	2	ECTS
ARTH.04.023	Prevention of HIV/AIDS and HIV Positive Patient	2	ECTS
ARTH.04.022	Principles of Sexuality Education	3	ECTS
ARFA.02.145	Seminars in Pharmaceutical Sciences I	1	ECTS
ARTH.04.024	Smoking and Health	1	ECTS
LOKT.01.017	Solutions	2	ECTS
ARSI.01.015	Spectacles, Contact Lenses and Refractive Surgery	1	ECTS
ARLA.01.033	Why and to Which Factors We are Allergic?	2	ECTS
2.2 Second course elective subjects (5 ECTS)			
ARBK.01.021	Basic Knowledge for the Research in Medical Biochemistry (I)	2	ECTS
ARMP.03.019	Basic Research in Pathophysiology I	6	ECTS
ARMP.03.020	Basic Research in Pathophysiology II	6	ECTS
ARFA.02.080	Exercises and Problems in Pharmaceutical Analysis	1	ECTS
ARLA.01.034	Foetal and Neonatal Physiology and Behaviour, Breastfeeding	2	ECTS
ARSK.00.009	Gerontology. Introduction (web-based)	3	ECTS
ARFA.02.138	Interdisciplinary Seminars in Pharmacy	2	ECTS
ARFS.01.005	Neurophysiology of Pain	2	ECTS
ARFA.01.106	Pharmacist in pharmacy system	2	ECTS
ARTH.04.023	Prevention of HIV/AIDS and HIV Positive Patient	2	ECTS
ARTH.04.022	Principles of Sexuality Education	3	ECTS
ARFA.02.019	Propaedeutical Training	3	ECTS
ARFA.02.081	Radiopharmaceuticals	1	ECTS
ARFA.02.145	Seminars in Pharmaceutical Sciences I	1	ECTS
ARTH.04.024	Smoking and Health	1	ECTS
ARSI.01.015	Spectacles, Contact Lenses and Refractive Surgery	1	ECTS
ARFA.02.128	Student Research in Pharmacy I	3	ECTS
ARFA.02.135	Student Research in Pharmacy II	6	ECTS
ARLA.01.033	Why and to Which Factors We are Allergic?	2	ECTS
2.3 Third course elective subjects (5 ECTS)			
ARBK.01.035	Basic Knowledge for the Research in Medical Biochemistry (II)	5	ECTS
ARMP.03.019	Basic Research in Pathophysiology I	6	ECTS
ARMP.03.020	Basic Research in Pathophysiology II	6	ECTS
ARFA.02.124	Chemistry of Vitamins	2	ECTS
ARTH.01.080	Environmental and Occupational Toxicology	3	ECTS
ARFA.02.080	Exercises and Problems in Pharmaceutical Analysis	1	ECTS
ARLA.01.034	Foetal and Neonatal Physiology and Behaviour, Breastfeeding	2	ECTS
ARSK.00.009	Gerontology. Introduction (web-based)	3	ECTS
ARFA.02.126	Granulation and Tableting Technology	2	ECTS
ARTH.04.018	Health Promotion	2	ECTS
ARFA.02.138	Interdisciplinary Seminars in Pharmacy	2	ECTS
ARFS.01.005	Neurophysiology of Pain	2	ECTS
ARMP.03.025	Pathophysiology of Stress	1.5	ECTS
ARFA.01.106	Pharmacist in pharmacy system	2	ECTS
ARTH.04.023	Prevention of HIV/AIDS and HIV Positive Patient	2	ECTS
ARTH.04.022	Principles of Sexuality Education	3	ECTS
ARFA.02.081	Radiopharmaceuticals	1	ECTS
ARFA.02.145	Seminars in Pharmaceutical Sciences I	1	ECTS
ARTH.04.024	Smoking and Health	1	ECTS
ARSI.01.015	Spectacles, Contact Lenses and Refractive Surgery	1	ECTS
ARFA.02.128	Student Research in Pharmacy I	3	ECTS
ARFA.02.135	Student Research in Pharmacy II	6	ECTS
ARFA.02.130	Student Research in Pharmacy III	6	ECTS

Table A1. *Cont.*

Pharmacy (300 ECTS)			
ARFA.02.133	Student Research in Pharmacy IV	6	ECTS
ARFA.02.015	Synthesis of Active Substances	2	ECTS
ARFA.02.140	Vibrational Spectroscopy- Different Applications in Pharmaceutical Drug Development	1	ECTS
ARTH.01.014	Water and Health	2	ECTS
ARLA.01.033	Why and to Which Factors We are Allergic?	2	ECTS
ARTH.01.040	Work Stress and Health	2	ECTS
2.4 Fourth course elective subjects (6 ECTS)			
AROT.00.030	Andragogy and Higher Education	3	ECTS
AROT.00.033	Applications of Developmental Psychology in Nursing	3	ECTS
ARMP.03.019	Basic Research in Pathophysiology I	6	ECTS
ARMP.03.020	Basic Research in Pathophysiology II	6	ECTS
ARTH.01.080	Environmental and Occupational Toxicology	3	ECTS
ARFA.02.080	Exercises and Problems in Pharmaceutical Analysis	1	ECTS
ARLA.01.034	Foetal and Neonatal Physiology and Behaviour, Breastfeeding	2	ECTS
ARSK.00.009	Gerontology. Introduction (web-based)	3	ECTS
ARFA.02.126	Granulation and Tableting Technology	2	ECTS
AROT.00.036	Health Care System and Policy for Nursing Managers	3	ECTS
ARTH.04.018	Health Promotion	2	ECTS
ARFA.02.138	Interdisciplinary Seminars in Pharmacy	2	ECTS
ARAR.00.001	Medical Law	2	ECTS
ARFA.02.134	Minimally Invasive Medical Technology	2	ECTS
ARFS.01.005	Neurophysiology of Pain	2	ECTS
ARFA.02.132	Pharmaceutical Film and Nano-coatings	2	ECTS
ARFA.02.141	Pharmaceutical nanotechnology	4	ECTS
ARFA.01.106	Pharmacist in pharmacy system	2	ECTS
AROT.01.013	Planning and Designing of Developmental Projects in Nursing	3	ECTS
ARTH.04.023	Prevention of HIV/AIDS and HIV Positive Patient	2	ECTS
ARTH.04.022	Principles of Sexuality Education	3	ECTS
ARFA.02.081	Radiopharmaceuticals	1	ECTS
ARFA.02.145	Seminars in Pharmaceutical Sciences I	1	ECTS
ARTH.04.024	Smoking and Health	1	ECTS
ARFA.01.060	Social Pharmacy in the Professional Literature and Internet	2	ECTS
ARSI.01.015	Spectacles, Contact Lenses and Refractive Surgery	1	ECTS
ARFA.02.135	Student Research in Pharmacy II	6	ECTS
ARFA.02.130	Student Research in Pharmacy III	6	ECTS
ARFA.02.133	Student Research in Pharmacy IV	6	ECTS
ARFA.02.137	Student Research in Pharmacy V	6	ECTS
ARFA.02.015	Synthesis of Active Substances	2	ECTS
ARSK.00.027	Vaccine and Immunization Education	3	ECTS
ARFA.02.140	Vibrational Spectroscopy- Different Applications in Pharmaceutical Drug Development	1	ECTS
ARTH.01.014	Water and Health	2	ECTS
ARLA.01.033	Why and to Which Factors We are Allergic?	2	ECTS
ARTH.01.040	Work Stress and Health	2	ECTS
3. Pharmacy Practice (37 ECTS)			
ARFA.02.071	Pharmacy Practice	37	ECTS
4. Final Exam (5 ECTS)			
ARFA.02.060	Graduation Examination	5	ECTS
5. Optional courses (12 ECTS)			

Appendix B

Table A2. The European pharmacy competences framework.

	Domains and compenetnes
	Domain 1: Personal competences—learning and knowledge
1	Ability to identify learning needs and to learn independently (including continuous professional development, CPD).
2	Ability to apply logic to problem solving.
3	Ability to critically appraise relevant knowledge and to summarise the key points.
4	Ability to evaluate scientific data in line with current scientific and technological knowledge.
5	Ability to apply preclinical and clinical evidence-based medical science to pharmaceutical practice.
6	Ability to apply current knowledge of relevant legislation and codes of pharmacy practice.
	Domain 2: Personal competences—values
7	A professional approach to tasks and human relations.
8	Ability to maintain confidentiality.
9	Ability to take full responsibility for patient care.
10	Ability to inspire the confidence of others in one's actions and advise.
11	Knowledge of appropriate legislation and of ethics.
	Domain 3: Personal competences—communication and organisational skills
12	Ability to communicate effectively—both oral and written—in the locally relevant language.
13	Ability to effectively use information technology.
14	Ability to work effectively as part of a team.
15	Ability to implement general legal requirements that impact upon the practice of pharmacy (e.g., health and safety legislation, employment law).
16	Ability to contribute to the training of staff.
17	Ability to manage risk and quality of service issues.
18	Ability to identify the need for new services.
19	Ability to understand a business environment and develop entrepreneurship.
	Domain 4: Personal competences—research and industrial pharmacy
20	Knowledge of design, synthesis, isolation, characterisation and biological evaluation of active substances.
21	Knowledge of good manufacturing practice and of good laboratory practice.
22	Knowledge of European directives on qualified persons.
23	Knowledge of drug registration, licensing and marketing.
24	Knowledge of the importance of research in pharmaceutical development and practice.
	Domain 5: Patient care competences—patient consultation and assessment
25	Ability to interpret basic medical laboratory tests.
26	Ability to perform appropriate diagnostic tests e.g., measurement of blood pressure or blood sugar.
27	Ability to recognise when referral to another member of the healthcare team is needed.
	Domain 6: Patient care competences—need for drug treatment
28	Ability to retrieve and interpret information on the patient's clinical background.
29	Ability to compile and interpret a comprehensive drug history for an individual patient.
30	Ability to identify non-adherence to medicine therapy and make an appropriate intervention.
31	Ability to advise to physicians on the appropriateness of prescribed medicines and—in some cases—to prescribe medication.
	Domain 7: Patient care competences—drug interactions
32	Ability to identify and prioritise drug-drug interactions and advise appropriate changes to medication.
33	Ability to identify and prioritise drug-patient interactions, including those that prevent or require the use of a specific drug, based on pharmaco-genetics, and advise on appropriate changes to medication.

Table A2. *Cont.*

	Domains and compenetnes
34	Ability to identify and prioritise drug-disease interactions (e.g., NSAIDs in heart failure) and advise on appropriate changes to medication.
	Domain 8: Patient care competences—drug dose and formulation
35	Knowledge of the bio-pharmaceutical, pharmacodynamic and pharmacokinetic activity of a substance in the body.
36	Ability to recommend interchangeability of drugs based on in-depth understanding and knowledge of bioequivalence, bio-similarity and therapeutic equivalence of drugs.
37	Ability to undertake a critical evaluation of a prescription ensuring that it is clinically appropriate and legally valid.
38	Knowledge of the supply chain of medicines thus ensuring timely flow of quality drug products to the patient.
39	Ability to manufacture medicinal products that are not commercially available.
	Domain 9: Patient care competences—patient education
40	Ability to promote public health in collaboration with other professionals within the healthcare system.
41	Ability to provide appropriate lifestyle advice to improve patient outcomes (e.g., advice on smoking, obesity, etc.).
42	Ability to use pharmaceutical knowledge and provide evidence-based advice on public health issues involving medicines.
	Domain 10: Patient care competences—provision of information and service
43	Ability to use effective consultations to identify the patient's need for information.
44	Ability to provide accurate and appropriate information on prescription medicines.
45	Ability to provide evidence-based support for patients in selection and use of non- prescription medicines.
	Domain 11: Patient care competences—monitoring of drug therapy
46	Ability to identify and prioritise problems in the management of medicines in a timely and effective manner and so ensure patient safety.
47	Ability to monitor and report Adverse Drug Events and Adverse Drug Reactions (ADEs and ADRs) to all concerned, in a timely manner, and in accordance with current regulatory guidelines on Good Pharmacovigilance Practices (GVPs).
48	Ability to undertake a critical evaluation of prescribed medicines to confirm that current clinical guidelines are appropriately applied.
49	Ability to monitor patient care outcomes to optimise treatment in collaboration with the prescriber.
50	Ability to contribute to the cost effectiveness of treatment by collection and analysis of data on medicines use.

References

1. Medical Faculty, University of Tartu, Estonia. Available online: http://meditsiiniteadused.ut.ee/en (accessed on 19 December 2016).
2. Sepp, K.; Lenbaum, K.; Laius, O.; Viidalepp, A.; Volmer, D. The "Quality guidelines for community pharmacy services"—A tool for harminozation of community pharmacy practice in Estonia. *Int. J. Clin. Pharm.* **2015**, *10* (Suppl. 1), 33.
3. Tallinn Healthcare College. Available online: http://www.ttk.ee/en/assistant-pharmacist-0 (accessed on 27 December 2016).
4. Medicinal Products Act. Available online: https://www.riigiteataja.ee/en/eli/ee/525112013005/consolide/current (accessed on 27 December 2016).
5. Directive 2005/36/EC of the European Parliament and of the Council on the recognition of professional qualifications. *Off. J. Eur. Union* **2005**, *L255*, 22–142. Available online: http://eur-lex.europa.eu/legal-content/en/TXT/?uri=CELEX%3A32005L0036 (accessed on 28 March 2017).
6. Directive 2013/55/EU of the European Parliament and of the Council amending Directive 2005/36/EC on the recognition of professional qualifications. *Off. J. Eur. Union* **2013**, *354*, 132–170. Available online: http://eur-lex.europa.eu/legal-content/EN/ALL/?uri=celex%3A32013L0055 (accessed on 28 March 2017).

7. Medicine Study Programme Group. *Self-Evaluation Report*; Department of Pharmacy, University of Tartu: Tartu, Estonia, 2014.

8. Atkinson, J.; Rombaut, B. The 2011 PHARMINE report on pharmacy and pharmacy education in the European Union. *Pharm. Pract. (Internet)* **2011**, *9*, 169–187. [CrossRef]

9. Quality Guidelines for Community Pharmacy Services. Available online: http://www.ravimiamet. ee/sites/default/files/documents/publications/apteegiteenuse_kvaliteedijuhis_2016/apteegiteenuse_ kvaliteedijuhis_2016.html#/0 (accessed on 10 December 2016).

10. Good Hospital Pharmacy Practice. Available online: http://media.voog.com/0000/0003/1027/files/16.02. 18%20-%20Eesti%20haiglafarmaatsia%20head%20tavad_Kodulehele.pdf (accessed on 10 December 2016).

11. CoDEG (Competency Development and Evaluation Group). General Level Practice. Available online: http://www.codeg.org/frameworks/general-level-practice (accessed on 16 December 2016).

12. Accreditation Council for Pharmacy Education. ACPE Open Forum: Accreditation Standards 2016. Available online: http://www.aacp.org/governance/SIGS/assessment/Assessment%20Docs/AACP% 202014%20Interim%20Meeting%20%20presentation%20-%20ACPE%20Standards%202016.pdf (accessed on 16 December 2016).

13. Stupans, I.; McAllister, S.; Clifford, R.; Hughes, J.; Krass, I.; March, G.; Owen, S.; Woulfeg, J. Nationwide collaborative development of learning outcomes and exemplar standards for Australian pharmacy programmes. *Int. J. Pharm. Pract.* **2015**, *23*, 283–291. [CrossRef] [PubMed]

14. FIP/WHO. International Pharmaceutical Federation—World Health Organisation: Standards for Quality of Pharmacy Services. Available online: https://www.fip.org (accessed on 16 December 2016).

15. Antoniou, S.; Webb, D.G.; Mcrobbie, D.; Davies, J.G.; Bates, I.P. A controlled study of the general level framework: Results of the South of England Competency Study. *Pharm. Educ.* **2005**, *5*, 201–207. [CrossRef]

16. Coombes, I.; Avent, M.; Cardiff, L.; Bettenay, K.; Coombes, J.; Whitfield, K.; Stokes, J.; Davies, G.; Bates, I. Improvement in pharmacist's performance facilitated by an adapted competency-based general level framework. *J. Pharm. Pract. Res.* **2010**, *40*, 111–118. [CrossRef]

17. AFPC. Educational Outcomes for First Professional Degree Programs in Pharmacy (Entry to Practice Pharmacy Programs) in Canada. Association of Faculties of Pharmacy of Canada (AFPC): Vancouver, 2010. Available online: www.afpc.info/sites/default/files/AFPC%20Educational%20Outcomes.pdf (accessed on 16 December 16 2016).

18. GPhC. Standards for the Initial Education and Training of Pharmacists. General Pharmaceutical Council (GPhC), 2011. Available online: www.pharmacyregulation.org/sites/default/files/GPhC_Future_ Pharmacists.pdf (accessed on 16 December 2016).

19. NCSF. National Competency Standards Framework for Pharmacists in Australia, Pharmaceutical Society for Australia (PSA), 2010. Available online: www.psa.org.au/downloads/standards/competency-standards-complete.pdf (accessed on 16 December 2016).

20. Atkinson, J.; Rombaut, B.; Sánchez Pozo, A.; Rekkas, D.; Veski, P.; Hirvonen, J.; Bozic, B.; Skowron, A.; Mircioiu, C.; Marcincal, A.; Wilson, K. Systems for Quality Assurance in Pharmacy Education and Training in the European Union. *Pharmacy* **2014**, *2*, 17–26. [CrossRef]

21. Atkinson, J.; De Paepe, K.; Sánchez Pozo, A.; Rekkas, D.; Volmer, D.; Hirvonen, J.; Bozic, B.; Skowron, A.; Mircioiu, C.; Marcincal, A.; et al. The PHAR-QA Project: Competency Framework for Pharmacy Practice—First Steps, the Results of the European Network Delphi Round 1. *Pharmacy* **2015**, *3*, 307–329. [CrossRef]

22. Atkinson, J.; De Paepe, K.; Sánchez Pozo, A.; Rekkas, D.; Volmer, D.; Hirvonen, J.; Bozic, B.; Skowron, A.; Mircioiu, C.; Marcincal, A.; et al. The Second Round of the PHAR-QA Survey of Competences for Pharmacy Practice. *Pharmacy* **2016**, *4*, 27. [CrossRef]

23. Pharmacist Competency Framework & Domain-specific Frame of Reference for the Netherlands. Available online: https://www.knmp.nl/downloads/pharmacist-competency-frameworkandDSFR-Netherlands.pdf (accessed on 19 February 2017).

24. Quality Assessment of the Study Programme Group Medicine at the University of Tartu, Estonia. Available online: http://ekka.archimedes.ee/wp-content/uploads/TU-meditsiin-assessment-report.pdf (accessed on 15 December 2016).

25. Occupational Qualification Standards for Pharmacists and Assistant Pharmacists were Approved in Estonia. Available online: http://www.kutsekoda.ee/et/kutseregister/kutsestandardid/10622084 (accessed on 18 December 2016).
26. Good Practice of Learning. Available online: http://www.tyye.ee/en/good-practice-learning (accessed on 27 December 2016).
27. Good Practice of Teaching. Available online: http://www.ut.ee/en/search/google/good%20practice%20of%20teaching (accessed on 27 December 2016).

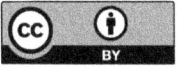

pharmacy

MDPI

Article

Curriculum Mapping of the Master's Program in Pharmacy in Slovenia with the PHAR-QA Competency Framework

Tanja Gmeiner, Nejc Horvat, Mitja Kos, Aleš Obreza, Tomaž Vovk, Iztok Grabnar and Borut Božič *

Faculty of Pharmacy, University of Ljubljana, Askerčeva 7, 1000 Ljubljana, Slovenia;
Tanja.Gmeiner@ffa.uni-lj.si (T.G.); Nejc.Horvat@ffa.uni-lj.si (N.H.); Mitja.Kos@ffa.uni-lj.si (M.K.);
Ales.Obreza@ffa.uni-lj.si (A.O.); Tomaz.Vovk@ffa.uni-lj.si (T.V.); Iztok.Grabnar@ffa.uni-lj.si (I.G.)
* Correspondence: borut.bozic@ffa.uni-lj.si; Tel.: +386-1-4769-501

Academic Editor: Jeffrey Atkinson
Received: 29 December 2016; Accepted: 22 April 2017; Published: 2 May 2017

Abstract: This article presents the results of mapping the Slovenian pharmacy curriculum to evaluate the adequacy of the recently developed and validated European Pharmacy Competences Framework (EPCF). The mapping was carried out and evaluated progressively by seven members of the teaching staff at the University of Ljubljana's Faculty of Pharmacy. Consensus was achieved by using a two-round modified Delphi technique to evaluate the coverage of competences in the current curriculum. The preliminary results of the curriculum mapping showed that all of the competences as defined by the EPCF are covered in Ljubljana's academic program. However, because most EPCF competences cover healthcare-oriented pharmacy practice, a lack of competences was observed for the drug development and production perspectives. Both of these perspectives are important because a pharmacist is (or should be) responsible for the entire process, from the development and production of medicines to pharmaceutical care in contact with patients. Nevertheless, Ljubljana's graduates are employed in both of these pharmaceutical professions in comparable proportions. The Delphi study revealed that the majority of differences in scoring arise from different perspectives on the pharmacy profession (e.g., community, hospital, industrial, etc.). Nevertheless, it can be concluded that curriculum mapping using the EPCF is very useful for evaluating and recognizing weak and strong points of the curriculum. However, the competences of the framework should address various fields of the pharmacist's profession in a more balanced way.

Keywords: pharmacy education; competences; curriculum mapping; community pharmacy; industrial pharmacy; clinical pharmacy; Delphi study; quality assurance; European framework

1. Introduction

Traditional universities structured programs with a defined number of courses, exams, and contact hours. It was up to the teachers to know what students needed in order to graduate from the university. The system was rather clear and worked smoothly. The majority of older pharmacists received their degrees through education structured in this way, and the pharmacy profession developed well, even excellently. Three independent factors resulted in a need to change this mindset in order to introduce competence-oriented curricula: (a) a significantly greater amount of information (not necessarily knowledge), (b) a shorter half-life of research-based knowledge, and (c) an increasing number of universities due to drastic changes in the expectations of the general population. Namely, only 2% of the population was expected to participate in higher education in the 19th century, compared to the European trend of the 21st century, in which 40% of the population is expected to participate in higher education. The change is not an issue of quantity alone, but also a question of quality. To meet the needs and expectations of society, curricula need to be reoriented from a structured mode to a competence-oriented mode [1,2].

Pharmacy education has deep roots in Slovenia. The principles of quality work in the pharmaceutical profession were introduced as early as in the 17th and 18th centuries. In 1710, a Pharmaceutical code was introduced for the Duchy of Carniola. Under the Illyrian Provinces at the beginning of the 19th century, pharmacy was taught through *materia medica* and pharmaceutical chemistry as the main subjects at the Central school in Ljubljana. Competences in pharmaceutical technology were built through traineeship at community or hospital pharmacies. University teaching of pharmacy was established in Ljubljana in the mid-20th century, with the first attempts in 1946 and 1955 as a two-year program, and starting in 1960 as a complete eight-semester program [3]. The development of undergraduate pharmacy education including clinical chemistry was based on the connection between research and practical applications in all fields of the pharmaceutical profession and science. The program was revamped several times, and it was extended to a four-and-a-half-year program in the mid-1990s. To show the integrity of the competences obtained, the curricula included awarding a diploma for individual student research work from the very beginning. After receiving their degrees, the graduates were employed as healthcare professionals (at community pharmacies, hospital pharmacies, and medical laboratories), researchers (in the public or private sector), in the pharmaceutical industry (in all four sectors: research and development, production, quality assurance, and marketing and sales), as teachers (at high schools and universities), or as professionals in pharmaceutical legislation. For employment, graduates needed to complete a probationary period and pass the final state exam. Several minor changes in the probation period based on future employers' needs were introduced before the program was harmonized according to European directives in 2004, when Slovenia entered the EU. Six months of traineeship in a pharmacy was included in the curriculum in the last semester of the five-year program [4]. Finally, the program was revamped and improved as a part of the Bologna process to a 10-semester uniform masters program: eight semesters of lectures, seminars, lab work, and other activities, one semester (6 months) of traineeship in pharmacies, and one semester of individual research work for the master's thesis. The state exam for pharmacists as healthcare professionals was integrated into the last semester, and was completed with a public defense of the master's thesis. The program was accredited by the National Agency for Quality in Higher Education in 2007 and was reaccredited in 2015 [5].

Several stakeholders were involved in the process of reform and accreditation through roundtables, workshops, meetings, written opinions, and other means. These included teachers from the university faculties involved (pharmacy, chemistry, medicine, mathematics, and physics), students (through the student counsel and the pharmacy students association), graduates, professional societies and chambers (the Slovenian Pharmaceutical Society, the Slovenian Chamber of Pharmacies, and the Slovenian Chamber of Laboratory Medicine), potential employers such as directors of community and hospital pharmacies, generic and innovative industry, and regulators (the Ministry of Health, and the Public Agency for Medicinal Products and Medical Devices). With this approach, we addressed recommendations by High Level Group on the Modernization of Higher Education, published in 2013 [1]. Namely, the program provides competences for employment in community pharmacies, hospital pharmacies, the pharmaceutical industry, medical laboratories, research laboratories, legislation, and education [6]. In some areas, an additional three or four years of specialization (as training) is necessary for special areas of the pharmacy profession, such as specializations in clinical pharmacy, medical design, medical testing, clinical chemistry, and radiopharmacy. Doctoral study is open after a degree in several fields, such as pharmacy, clinical chemistry and laboratory medicine, toxicology, biochemistry and molecular biology, and genetics [7].

The master's program in pharmacy was designed for the first-day-of-job-pharmacist; that is, for novices or beginners with limited experience [8] to be able to work autonomously. During the education process, competences are built from lower to higher levels, and therefore horizontal and vertical course linkages are very important. The primary objective of the Faculty of Pharmacy is to develop scientifically and professionally qualified, high-quality graduates familiar with ethical principles that autonomously carry out demanding tasks in community and hospital pharmacies, in all fields of the pharmaceutical industry, in clinical laboratories and laboratory medicine, laboratories for drug control and analysis, research institutions, educational organizations, state bodies, and wherever the work and presence of a pharmacist is required to increase health safety [9]. The faculty's commitment to quality teaching and research has been shown through many activities, including participation in projects initiated by EAFP [10], such as Pharmacy Education in Europe (Pharmine) and Quality Assurance in European Pharmacy Education and Training (PHAR-QA).

The European Commission has funded the international project PHAR-QA [11] to produce a consensual, harmonized framework of competences for pharmacy practice across Europe. This framework is intended to be used as a base for a QA system for evaluating university pharmacy education and training at the institutional, national, and/or European levels [12]. The second round of the PHAR-QA survey of competences for pharmacy practice in Europe was completed in 2016 [13].

The aim of this study was to evaluate the usefulness of the framework developed for pharmaceutical competences as a tool for mapping the master's pharmacy curricula by matching the existing curriculum of the master's program in pharmacy in Slovenia to the framework.

2. Materials and Methods

A team of seven members of the teaching staff in the integrated master's program in pharmacy [6] at the University of Ljubljana's Faculty of Pharmacy was involved in curriculum mapping. Two members of the team have previously been involved in the PHAR-QA project [11]; three members are responsible for coordinating the master's program, international student exchange, and traineeship as part of undergraduate study; and four members of the team are also members of the faculty management. The mapping was carried out and evaluated progressively, as indicated.

Step 1: A Microsoft Excel file was generated composing a matrix of 50 European Pharmacy Competences Framework (EPCF) competences [13] versus 60 courses in the master's curriculum. For greater transparency of the file, clusters are separated into individual worksheets and the competences within each cluster are listed in the y-axis. Courses were listed in a "drop-down" form for each year of the program in the x-axis (Figure 1).

Step 2: Primary mapping was done by a single member of the team, who copy-pasted the competences as described in the master's curriculum from each course individually based on personal assessment of the matching. In cases where competences were defined more generically (covering multiple competences), they were mapped in two or more PHAR-QA competences. For example: the competence from the program "Students acquire basic knowledge about drug action within an organism and the organism's reaction upon exposure to drug(s)" was mapped in "(29) Ability to compile and interpret a comprehensive drug history for an individual patient," "(34) Ability to identify and prioritize drug-disease interactions (e.g., NSAIDs in heart failure) and advise on appropriate changes to medication," and "(35) Knowledge of the bio-pharmaceutical, pharmacodynamic, and pharmacokinetic activity of a substance in the body."

If the description was too general, such as: "Development of competences and skills of using knowledge in a particular professional area," or not listed in the EPCF list, the faculty's competence was listed in a separate worksheet.

Step 3: The result of the primary mapping was individually evaluated and revised by the coordinator of the master's program, coordinator of the international student exchange, and coordinator of the traineeship. The revision was made based on their thorough knowledge of the course syllabuses.

Step 4: The final review of the mapping process and evaluation was made by all seven members of the team. Special attention was paid to:

- Competences absent from the curriculum;
- The number of times each competence was addressed in the curriculum;
- Building competences through teaching from lower to higher levels;
- Dedicated time and ECTS credits planned in the curriculum for teaching to build individual competences.

Step 5: Gaps and inconsistences in the curriculum and EPCF list were identified.

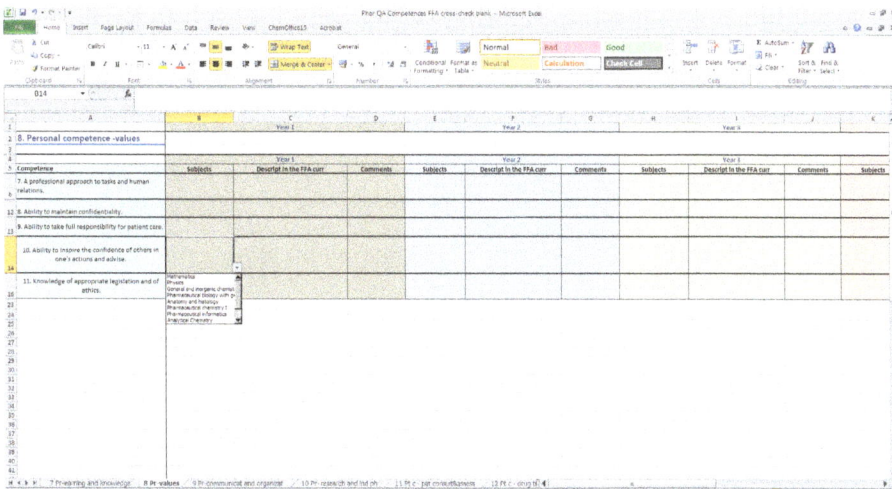

Figure 1. Screen-shot of the worksheet of a Microsoft Excel file generated for curricula mapping. Each worksheet includes one cluster of competences as defined by the Quality Assurance in European Pharmacy Education and Training (PHAR-QA) project (11). The competences within the clusters are listed in the ordinate. The courses in the master's curriculum are arranged in "drop-down" form, matching the individual year of the master's program in the abscissa.

The level of agreement of scores among individual evaluators participating in the study was assessed using the Delphi methodology [14,15]. A Delphi consensus panel was run with the aim of evaluating coverage of competences as defined by the PharQA framework in the current master's curriculum. The Delphi expert panel included four independent ratings performed by two individuals and two teams with two evaluators working together. The evaluators were six faculty professors that have insight into the pharmacy curriculum. The Delphi study consisted of two rounds. In the first round, panelists rated the coverage of the competences in the curriculum. Coverage was scored using the following five-point Likert-type scale: 0 = not covered at all, 1 = poor, 2 = fair, 3 = good, 4 = very good. Consensus on the coverage of competences was defined as the range of individual scores (Max–Min) being one or less. The panelists were also asked to provide comments on the clarity and their understanding of competences.

After the first round, the expert panel members met for a roundtable discussion. The results of the first round were presented and the panelists discussed the items for which consensus on coverage had not been attained and clarified the differences in ratings. In the second round, the panelists once again rated the coverage of competences, taking into account the roundtable discussion, the median of the panelists' answers, and the response distribution from the first round. Consensus was defined as the range being one or less.

3. Results

The starting point was the EPCF list of competences, and whether and where a particular competence is present in the curriculum was checked. The Slovenian pharmacy master's curriculum consists of 60 courses (subjects) in a 10-semester uniform program including a six-month traineeship in pharmacy, individual research work, and a master's thesis defense. The preliminary results of the competence mapping are presented in Table 1. The numbering of the competences in the table is consistent with the numbering in the PHAR-QA project [13], in which the first six questions address the profile of the respondents (age, duration of practice, country of residence, and current occupation) and were not included in the mapping process. The questions in clusters 7–16 are reflected in 60 competences for pharmacy practice across Europe: clusters 7–10 cover personal competences, and clusters 11–17 cover patient care competences.

Table 1. Results of curriculum mapping of the competences in the Slovenian master's program in pharmacy. Subjects are arranged by program years, and clusters of competences are defined by PHAR-QA. The numbers indicate how many competences from each cluster are defined in each of the subjects. Subjects are listed in alphabetical order by each year of the program.

Subject	7- Learning and Knowledge	8- Values	9- Communication and 9- Organisational 9- Skills	10- Research and Industrial Pharmacy	11- Patient Consultation and Assessment	12- Need for Drug Treatment	13- Drug Interactions	14- Drug dose and Formulation	15- Patient Education	16- Provision of Information and Service	17- Monitoring of Drug therapy	ECTS	Sum of All Competences Per Subject
	Personal Competences				Patient Care Competences								
Year 1													
Analytical Chemistry	2	0	0	0	0	0	0	0	0	0	0	8	2
Anatomy and histology	0	0	0	0	0	1	0	0	0	0	0	8	1
General and inorganic chemistry	2	0	0	0	0	0	0	0	0	0	0	8	2
Introduction to pharmacy	1	4	0	2	0	0	0	0	0	0	0	3	7
Mathematics	1	0	0	0	0	0	0	0	0	0	0	7	1
Microbiology	0	0	0	0	1	1	0	0	0	0	0	4	2
Pharmaceutical biology with genetics	5	3	3	0	0	0	0	0	0	0	0	7	11
Pharmaceutical chemistry I	2	0	0	0	0	0	0	0	0	0	0	6	2
Pharmaceutical informatics	1	0	1	1	0	0	0	0	0	0	2	5	5
Physics	1	0	0	0	0	0	0	0	0	0	0	8	1
Year 2													
Organic chemistry	0	0	1	1	0	0	0	0	0	0	0	9	2
Pharmaceutical biochemistry	2	0	0	0	0	0	0	0	0	1	0	7	3
Pharmaceutical chemistry II	1	0	0	1	0	1	1	1	0	0	0	7	5
Pharmaceutical technology I	1	1	4	4	0	0	0	1	0	1	0	20	12
Physical chemistry	1	0	0	0	0	0	0	0	0	0	0	6	1
Physical pharmacy	0	0	0	1	0	0	0	0	0	0	0	5	1
Physiology	1	0	0	0	1	0	0	0	0	0	0	6	2
Year 3													
Cosmetology	1	0	0	1	0	0	0	0	0	0	0	5	2
Hospital Pharmacy	0	1	3	1	0	1	0	1	0	0	1	5	8
Immunology	2	0	1	0	0	1	0	0	0	0	0	5	4
Instrumental Analytical Methods in Pharmacy	1	0	0	0	0	0	0	0	0	0	0	5	1
Instrumental pharmaceutical analysis	1	0	1	1	0	0	0	0	0	0	0	4	3
Nutritional Supplements	2	2	3	0	0	0	0	0	0	1	0	5	8
Pathologic physiology	2	0	0	0	0	1	0	0	0	0	0	6	3

Table 1. *Cont.*

Cluster of Competences Subject	7-Learning and Knowledge	8-Values	9- Communication and 9-Organisational 9-Skills	10- Research and Industrial Pharmacy	11- Patient Consultation and Assessment	12- Need for Drug Treatment	13- Drug Interactions	14- Drug dose and Formulation	15- Patient Education	16- Provision of Information and Service	17- Monitoring of Drug therapy	ECTS	Sum of All Competences Per Subject
	Personal Competences				Patient Care Competences								
Year 3													
Pharmaceutical chemistry III	0	0	1	3	0	0	2	1	0	0	0	20	7
Pharmaceutical Marketing and Management	0	0	1	1	0	0	0	1	0	0	0	5	3
Pharmaceutical technology II	1	1	1	2	0	0	0	0	0	0	0	8	5
Pharmacoeconomics	0	0	2	0	0	0	0	0	0	0	1	5	3
Pharmacognosy I	2	2	3	0	0	0	0	0	0	1	0	9	8
Pharmacognosy II	2	2	3	1	0	0	0	1	0	0	0	4	9
Research methods in social Pharmacy	0	0	0	1	0	0	0	1	0	0	2	5	4
Social pharmacy	2	0	4	0	0	0	0	2	2	2	5	4	17
Year 4													
Analysis and supervision of medicinal products	2	0	0	4	0	0	0	0	0	0	0	8	6
Biochemistry of Cancer Development and Progression	1	1	0	0	0	0	0	0	0	0	0	5	2
Biopharmaceutical Evaluation of Pharmaceutical Forms	0	0	0	1	0	0	0	1	0	0	0	5	2
Biopharmaceutics with pharmacokinetics	0	0	0	2	0	1	2	2	0	0	0	9	7
Clinical chemistry	1	0	2	1	3	0	0	0	0	0	0	7	7
Clinical pharmacy	1	4	0	0	0	4	3	1	2	2	3	5	20
Design and Synthesis of Active Substances	1	0	0	1	0	0	0	1	0	0	0	5	3
Eutomers	0	0	0	2	0	0	0	1	0	0	0	5	3
Industrial pharmacy	1	0	0	4	0	0	0	0	0	0	0	5	5
Medicinal Products of alternative Medicine	3	2	2	0	0	0	0	0	0	0	0	5	7
Modified Release Pharmaceutical Forms	2	1	0	1	0	0	0	0	0	0	0	5	4
Pharmaceutical biotechnology	2	2	2	3	0	0	0	2	0	0	0	6	11
Pharmaceutical Engineering	0	0	0	1	0	0	0	0	0	0	0	5	1
Pharmacogenomics and Genetic Medicines	1	1	1	2	0	0	1	0	0	0	0	5	6
Pharmacology	1	0	0	0	0	1	2	2	0	0	0	5	6
Phytopharmaceuticals	2	2	0	0	0	0	0	0	0	1	0	5	5
Psychotropic substances and Abuse of Medicinal Products	1	0	0	0	0	2	0	0	0	0	0	5	3
Quality of Medicinal Products	0	0	0	3	0	0	0	0	0	0	0	5	3
Selected Methods of Pharmaceutical Analysis	1	0	0	0	0	0	0	0	0	0	0	5	1
Selected Topics in Clinical Biochemistry	0	0	0	0	2	0	0	0	0	0	0	5	2
Selected Topics in Pharmaceutical Biotechnology	1	2	3	2	0	0	0	1	0	0	0	5	9
Stability of medicinals	1	0	0	1	0	0	0	0	0	0	0	5	2
The Use of Genetic and Cellular Testing in Biomedicine and Pharmacy	0	1	1	0	1	0	1	0	0	0	0	5	4
Toxicological chemistry	1	0	0	1	0	1	0	0	0	0	0	5	3
Year 5													
Individual research work for master's thesis	1	1	2	0	0	0	0	0	0	0	0	25	4
Master's thesis defence	2	1	2	0	0	0	0	0	0	0	0	5	5
Traineeship	3	4	7	2	1	3	3	4	3	3	3	30	36
Sum	68	39	58	57	9	18	15	25	7	13	17	410	

Legend:

1st year of study
2nd year of study
3rd year of study
4th year of study
5th year of study

All competences as defined by the EPCF are covered in our master's curriculum, although their distribution among subjects and across program years is not balanced. During the first two years of the master's program, in which the curriculum contains typically basic subjects in the natural sciences, personal competences from clusters 7 through 11 are predominantly covered, especially those dealing with abilities to learn independently and apply logic to solve problems. Later in the program, competences from all groups are distributed more evenly. It is also evident that each subject addresses at least one EPCF competence.

The preliminary results are a rough estimate of how competences are covered in our curriculum. It was obvious that the description of competences in the curriculum was not sufficient for adequate scoring. Namely, some competences are addressed several times in a particular subject and it is not clear to what extent the competence is actually covered (i.e., mentioned, discussed, or elaborated). On the other hand, it is not possible to recognize progression in the level and sequence of student learning and performance through the program. For this reason, the evaluation was enhanced by using the Delphi approach.

Tables 2 and 3 present coverage of competence domains and individual competences in the first and second rounds of the Delphi study. Table 4 presents consensus building between the first and second rounds of the Delphi study.

Table 2. Coverage of competence domains as defined by the PHAR-QA framework in the Slovenian pharmacy curriculum. Results from both rounds of the Delphi study are presented as weighted medians of all competences in the domain. Coverage was scored using a five-point Likert-type scale: 0 = not covered at all, 1 = poor, 2 = fair, 3 = good, 4 = very good.

Domain	Coverage of the Competency Domain	
	1st Round Weighted Median	2nd Round Weighted Median
7. Personal competences: learning and knowledge.	3,4	3,4
8. Personal competences: values.	2,7	2,6
9. Personal competences: communication and organizational skills.	2,2	2,2
10. Personal competences: research and industrial pharmacy.	3,0	3,0
11. Patient care competences: patient consultation and assessment.	2,7	3,0
12. Patient care competences: need for drug treatment.	2,3	2,3
13. Patient care competences: drug interactions.	2,2	2,3
14. Patient care competences: drug dose and formulation.	3,3	3,2
15. Patient care competences: patient education.	2,0	2,0
16. Patient care competences: provision of information and service.	2,7	2,8
17. Patient care competences: monitoring of drug therapy.	2,0	2,0

Legend: An MS Excel three-color scale algorithm was used to present the results of the Delphi rounds, whereby the lowest value is presented in red, the highest in green, and the median in yellow.

Table 3. Coverage of individual competences as defined by the PHAR-QA framework in the Slovenian pharmacy curriculum. Results from both rounds of the Delphi study are presented. Coverage was scored using a five-point Likert-type scale: 0 = not covered at all, 1 = poor, 2 = fair, 3 = good, 4 = very good.

Competency Organised According to Domains	Coverage of Individual Competencies	
	1st Round Median (Min–Max)	2nd Round Median (Min–Max)
Domain: 7. Personal competences: learning and knowledge.		
1. Ability to identify learning needs and to learn independently (including continuous professional development (CPD).	3 (2–4)	3 (3–3)
2. Ability to apply logic to problem solving.	4 (4–4)	4 (4–4)
3. Ability to critically appraise relevant knowledge and to summarise the key points.	4 (3–4)	4 (3–4)
4. Ability to evaluate scientific data in line with current scientific and technological knowledge.	4 (3–4)	4 (4–4)

Table 3. *Cont.*

Competency Organised According to Domains	Coverage of Individual Competencies	
	1st Round Median (Min–Max)	2nd Round Median (Min–Max)
Domain: 7. Personal competences: learning and knowledge.		
5. Ability to apply preclinical and clinical evidence-based medical science to pharmaceutical practice.	3 (2–3)	3 (3–3)
6. Ability to apply current knowledge of relevant legislation and codes of pharmacy practice.	2,5 (2–4)	2,5 (2–3)
Domain: 8. Personal competences: values.		
1. A professional approach to tasks and human relations.	3 (2–4)	3 (3–4)
2. Ability to maintain confidentiality.	3 (2–4)	3 (3–3)
3. Ability to take full responsibility for patient care.	2 (1–2)	2 (1–2)
4. Ability to inspire the confidence of others in one's actions and advise.	2 (2–3)	2 (2–3)
5. Knowledge of appropriate legislation and of ethics.	3,5 (2–4)	3 (3–4)
Domain: 9. Personal competences: communication and organisational skills.		
1. Ability to communicate effectively—both oral and written—in the locally relevant language.	3 (3–4)	3 (3–4)
2. Ability to effectively use information technology.	2,5 (2–3)	2,5 (2–3)
3. Ability to work effectively as part of a team.	3 (2–4)	3 (3–3)
4. Ability to implement general legal requirements that impact upon the practice of pharmacy (e.g., health and safety legislation, employment law).	2,5 (2–4)	2,5 (2–3)
5. Ability to contribute to the training of staff.	1 (1–2)	1 (1–2)
6. Ability to manage risk and quality of service issues.	2 (1–2)	2 (1–2)
7. Ability to identify the need for new services.	1,5 (1–2)	1,5 (1–2)
8. Ability to understand a business environment and develop entrepreneurship.	2 (1–2)	2 (1–2)
Domain: 10. Personal competences: research and industrial pharmacy.		
1. Knowledge of design, synthesis, isolation, characterisation and biological evaluation of active substances.	4 (4–4)	4 (4–4)
2. Knowledge of good manufacturing practice and of good laboratory practice.	3 (3–4)	3 (3–4)
3. Knowledge of European directives on qualified persons.	1,5 (1–2)	1,5 (1–2)
4. Knowledge of drug registration, licensing and marketing.	3 (3–4)	3 (3–4)
5. Knowledge of the importance of research in pharmaceutical development and practice.	3,5 (2–4)	3,5 (3–4)
Domain: 11. Patient care competences: patient consultation and assessment.		
1. Ability to interpret basic medical laboratory tests.	4 (1–4)	4 (3–4)
2. Ability to perform appropriate diagnostic tests e.g., measurement of blood pressure or blood sugar.	1 (0–3)	2 (0–3)
3. Ability to recognise when referral to another member of the healthcare team is needed.	3 (2–3)	3 (2–3)
Domain: 12. Patient care competences: need for drug treatment.		
1. Ability to retrieve and interpret information on the patient's clinical background.	3 (1–3)	3 (3–3)
2. Ability to compile and interpret a comprehensive drug history for an individual patient.	2 (1–3)	2 (2–3)
3. Ability to identify non-adherence to medicine therapy and make an appropriate intervention.	2 (1–3)	2 (2–2)
4. Ability to advise to physicians on the appropriateness of prescribed medicines and—in some cases—to prescribe medication.	2 (1–3)	2 (1–2)
Domain: 13. Patient care competences: drug interactions.		
1. Ability to identify and prioritise drug-drug interactions and advise appropriate changes to medication.	3 (2–3)	3 (2–3)
2. Ability to identify and prioritise drug-patient interactions, including those that prevent or require the use of a specific drug, based on pharmaco-genetics, and advise on appropriate changes to medication.	1,5 (1–3)	2 (1–2)
3. Ability to identify and prioritise drug-disease interactions (e.g., NSAIDs in heart failure) and advise on appropriate changes to medication.	2 (1–2)	2 (1–2)
Domain: 14. Patient care competences: drug dose and formulation.		
1. Knowledge of the bio-pharmaceutical, pharmacodynamic and pharmacokinetic activity of a substance in the body.	4 (4–4)	4 (4–4)
2. Ability to recommend interchangeability of drugs based on in-depth understanding and knowledge of bioequivalence, bio-similarity and therapeutic equivalence of drugs.	3 (2–4)	3 (3–4)
3. Ability to undertake a critical evaluation of a prescription ensuring that it is clinically appropriate and legally valid.	2,5 (1–3)	2 (2–2)
4. Knowledge of the supply chain of medicines thus ensuring timely flow of quality drug products to the patient.	3 (2–3)	3 (2–3)
5. Ability to manufacture medicinal products that are not commercially available.	4 (3–4)	4 (3–4)

Table 3. *Cont.*

Competency Organised According to Domains	Coverage of Individual Competencies	
	1st Round Median (Min–Max)	**2nd Round** Median (Min–Max)
Domain: 15. Patient care competences: patient education.		
1. Ability to promote public health in collaboration with other professionals within the healthcare system.	2 (2–3)	2 (2–3)
2. Ability to provide appropriate lifestyle advice to improve patient outcomes (e.g., advice on smoking, obesity, etc.).	2 (2–3)	2 (2–3)
3. Ability to use pharmaceutical knowledge and provide evidence-based advice on public health issues involving medicines.	2 (2–3)	2 (2–3)
Domain: 16. Patient care competences: provision of information and service.		
1. Ability to use effective consultations to identify the patient's need for information.	2 (1–3)	2 (1–2)
2. Ability to provide accurate and appropriate information on prescription medicines.	3,5 (3–4)	3,5 (3–4)
3. Ability to provide evidence-based support for patients in selection and use of non-prescription medicines.	2,5 (2–4)	3 (3–4)
Domain: 17. Patient care competences: monitoring of drug therapy.		
1. Ability to identify and prioritise problems in the management of medicines in a timely and effective manner and so ensure patient safety.	2 (2–3)	2 (2–3)
2. Ability to monitor and report Adverse Drug Events and Adverse Drug Reactions (ADEs and ADRs) to all concerned, in a timely manner, and in accordance with current regulatory guidelines on Good Pharmacovigilance Practices (GVPs).	1,5 (1–2)	1,5 (1–2)
3. Ability to undertake a critical evaluation of prescribed medicines to confirm that current clinical guidelines are appropriately applied.	2,5 (2–3)	2,5 (2–3)
4. Ability to monitor patient care outcomes to optimise treatment in collaboration with the prescriber.	2 (1–2)	2 (1–2)
5. Ability to contribute to the cost effectiveness of treatment by collection and analysis of data on medicines use.	2 (1–3)	2 (2–3)

Legend: Results from the second round of the Delphi study that are shaded represent medians that changed from the first round of the Delphi study.

Table 4. Consensus building between the first and second rounds of the Delphi study. The frequency of ranges of individual scores (Max–Min) evaluating coverage of individual competences as defined by the PHAR-QA framework in the Slovenian pharmacy curriculum.

Range of Individual Scores (Max–Min)		2nd Round					
		0	1	2	3	4	Sum
	0	3	0	0	0	0	3
	1	2	25	0	0	0	27
1st	2	6	12	0	0	0	18
Round	3	0	1	0	1	0	2
	4	0	0	0	0	0	0
	Sum	11	38	0	1	0	50

4. Discussion

Evaluation was performed based on the curriculum [6]. The performance of the program (i.e., educational outcomes of the competences achieved) was not part of our study. The authors of this study are aware of different approaches in curriculum mapping. The final goal is to compare intended, perceived, and achieved competences as evaluated by students, graduates, teachers, and employers. Such mapping would be very useful in improving the program and its performance [16,17]. However, for preliminary mapping with the available resources, only the first step was realistic: mapping the curriculum delivered as written in the accreditation documents, expanded by evaluation of the competences present in the curricula as explained in the section Materials and Methods.

The master's program in pharmacy in Slovenia educates students for both aspects of pharmacy practice—working in health services and the pharmaceutical industry in approximately the same proportion—and most EPCF competences cover healthcare-oriented pharmacy practice; this is also reflected in the results of our evaluation. Personal competences are addressed with relatively higher frequencies due to the fact that the EPCF predominantly covers healthcare-oriented pharmacy competences. Namely, the definition of the pharmacy profession or pharmacy practice at the international level is not always clear [18]. There is no doubt that a pharmacist is a healthcare professional, but not only that. The pharmacist is "the university professional whose primary mission is the management and the exclusive responsibility for the formulation, preparation and the responsible dispensing of drugs to the population in addition to its inevitable participation in the protection of health and improvement of the quality of life" [19]. Several inconsistencies are evident regarding the pharmacist's role more broadly; that is, in the pharmaceutical industry in developing and producing medicines and in laboratory medicine. The master's program in Slovenia is designed to provide pharmacy competences within the healthcare system as well as the pharmaceutical industry, medical laboratories, research laboratories, legislation, and education. From this perspective, the PHAR-QA framework of competences does not sufficiently cover competences outside the healthcare system. Competences in drug development and production should be developed and included in greater detail.

Some definitions were found to be rather loose and/or ambiguous. For example, the competence "Knowledge of the importance of research in pharmaceutical development and practice" seems to be too general and is addressed by the majority of subjects in our curriculum. The members of the study team had difficulty understanding what the competence covers; it seems self-evident. The curriculum sets competences about research in pharmaceutical development and practice at a higher level according to Bloom's classification [20].

It was further observed that some competences are too broad, covering multiple competences. Some examples include the following: "Ability to undertake a critical evaluation of a prescription ensuring that it is clinically appropriate and legally valid" should distinguish competences of a clinical and legislative nature/origin; "Ability to advise physicians on the appropriateness of prescribed medicines and—in some cases—to prescribe medication" should distinguish counselling (i.e., advising) from taking actions (i.e., prescribing); and "Ability to identify non-adherence to medicine therapy and make an appropriate intervention" should distinguish the ability to recognize from the ability to intervene. The problem of scoring arises when two partial competences are not from the same origin and cannot be covered in the curriculum equally. For example, prescription of medicines by a pharmacist is not allowed in many EU countries, including Slovenia. Therefore it is unreasonable to include such competences in the national curriculum.

During the education process, competences are built from lower to higher levels according to Bloom's taxonomy: remember, understand, apply, analyze, evaluate, and create [21]. Not considering this, only courses at the top of the pillars are recognized as important for a particular competence whereas basic courses are overlooked. For example, the team had difficulty differentiating the following competences: "(7) Ability to apply current knowledge of relevant legislation and codes of pharmacy practice," "(8) Knowledge of appropriate legislation and of ethics," and "(9) Ability to implement general legal requirements that impact upon the practice of pharmacy"; it seems that different levels of Bloom's classification are being addressed inconsistently. To develop competences at higher levels (i.e., to be able to perform), several lower-level competences (i.e., knowledge and skills) should be adopted and included in the curriculum. Lower-level competences are usually written very generally, such as "development of skills" or "capability of practical application of knowledge," and are not linked to a specific field or competences. On the other hand, competence at the highest level, such as "Ability to use pharmaceutical knowledge and provide evidence-based advice on public health issues involving medicines," means that students have already built sufficient pharmaceutical knowledge, which should be addressed inside the curriculum as separate lower-level competences (knowledge and understanding).

The roundtable discussion of the Delphi study and further analysis of the results revealed that the majority of differences in scoring arise from different perspectives on the pharmacy profession (e.g., community, hospital, industrial, academic, laboratory medicine, or regulative); for example, "7. Personal competences: learning and knowledge. 6. Ability to apply current knowledge of relevant legislation and codes of pharmacy practice." Scoring pharmacy practice from a healthcare perspective yields different results than scoring pharmacy practice from a more general perspective, also covering industrial and regulatory aspects of the profession. Similarly, the competence "11. Patient care competences: patient consultation and assessment. 2. Ability to perform appropriate diagnostic tests, e.g., measurement of blood pressure or blood sugar" can be understood as graduates' ability to perform some basic diagnostic tests in community pharmacy, or graduates' ability to work in laboratory medicine (synonyms: clinical biochemistry, clinical biology) [22]. This is a common situation in Slovenia [23]. Different perspectives and understandings of competences as defined by PharQA were discussed in the roundtable, leading to more a balanced approach to evaluation among the panelists. This resulted in greater consensus in the second round of the Delphi evaluation process: the panelists reached consensus for 49 out of 50 competences.

Competences have to be designed to fit the first-day-of-job pharmacist [2,8]. From this perspective, it was found that some of the competences in the EPMF were rather too ambitious and require additional graduate training and/or specialization, as also discussed by Atkinson [13].

It can be concluded that curriculum mapping using EPMF is very useful for evaluating and recognizing weak and strong points of the curriculum. However, it must also be recognized that some additional improvement of the existing framework is needed. Namely, the competences of the framework should address various fields of the pharmacy profession in a more balanced way.

This study found the mapping process to be more complex than it seemed at the beginning. Not all of the pitfalls observed were addressed. For other mapping steps (e.g., perceived and achieved competences), some tuning differences in personal approaches would be necessary, and some kind of training would also be useful to support activities, which is in line with the recommendations of the European Commission [1] about teaching and learning improvement, and is also part of the Slovenian National Higher Education Program 2011–2020 [24].

Author Contributions: B.B. designed, constructed and leaded the process of curriculum mapping and analyzing. T.G. and B.B. prepared preliminary matrix courses/competences. B.B., A.O., I.G. and T.V. made preliminary mapping of the curriculum. T.G., N.H., M.K., A.O., T.V. and I.G. performed curriculum mapping. T.G., M.K., N.H. and A.O. analyzed data. B.B., M.K. and T.G. wrote the paper. All authors provided useful criticism and suggestions during paper writing.

Conflicts of Interest: The authors declare no conflict of interest.

References

1. High Level Group on the Modernisation of Higher Education. *Report to the European Commission on Improving the Quality of Teaching and Learning in Europe's Higher Education Institution*; Publications Office of the European Union: Luxembourg, 2013.
2. Božič, B. Competencies of the "first day of job" pharmacist, invited lecture. In *Abstract Book. II Congress of Pharmacists of Montenegro with the International Participation*; Potpara, Z., Ed.; UCG&FKCG: Budva, The Republic of Montenegro, 28–31 May 2015.
3. Božič, B.; Ribič, L. (Eds.) *Progress Report of the Faculty of Pharmacy for the Year 2012*; ULFFA: Ljubljana, Slovenia, 2013.
4. Directive 2005/36/EC of the European Parliament and of the Council of 7 September 2005 on the Recognition of Professional Qualifications. Available online: http://eur-lex.europa.eu/legal-content/en/TXT/?uri= CELEX%3A32005L0036 (accessed on 26 December 2016).
5. Slovenian Quality Assurance Agency for Higher Education. QA Procedures. Available online: http: //www.nakvis.si/en-GB/Content/Details/78 (accessed on 26 December 2016).
6. Uniform Master's Study Programme Pharmacy, University of Ljubljana, Faculty of Pharmacy, Slovenia. Available online: http://www.ffa.uni-lj.si/fileadmin/datoteke/Dekanat/Pravilniki/PROSPECTUS_ Pharmacy.pdf (accessed on 26 December 2016).
7. Interdisciplinary Doctoral Programme in Biomedicine, University of Ljubljana, Slovenia. Available online: http://www.ffa.uni-lj.si/fileadmin/datoteke/Dekanat/Studij/2013-14/Biomedicine_brochure_ en_20_3_2013.pdf (accessed on 26 December 2016).

8. Dreyfus, S.E.; Dreyfus, H.L. *A Five-Stage Model of the Mental Activities Involved in Directed Skill Acquisition*; Storming Media: Washington, DC, USA, 1980.
9. Božič, B.; Toth, B. (Eds.) *Report on the Achievements of the Faculty of Pharmacy for 2015*. Available online: http://www.ffa.uni-lj.si/en/faculty/presentation/reports (accessed on 28 December 2016).
10. European Association of Faculties of Pharmacy. Available online: http://eafponline.eu/euprojects/ (accessed on 26 December 2016).
11. The PHAR-QA Project: Quality Assurance in European Pharmacy Education and Training. Available online: http://www.phar-qa.eu/ (accessed on 26 December 2016).
12. Atkinson, J.; Rombaut, B.; Sanchez-Pozo, A.; Rekkas, D.; Veski, P.; Hirvonen, J.; Bozic, B.; Skowron, A.; Mirciou, C. A description of the European pharmacy education and training quality assurance project. *Pharmacy* **2013**, *1*, 3–7. [CrossRef]
13. Atkinson, J.; de Paepe, K.; Sánchez Pozo, A.; Rekkas, D.; Volmer, D.; Hirvonen, J.; Bozic, B.; Skowron, A.; Mircioiu, C.; Marcincal, A.; et al. The second round of the PHAR-QA survey of competences for pharmacy practice. *Pharmacy* **2016**, *4*, 27. [CrossRef]
14. Hsu, C.C.; Sandford, B.A. The Delphi Technique: Making Sense of Consensus. *Pract. Assess. Res. Eval.* **2007**, *12*, 1–8.
15. Atkinson, J.; de Paepe, K.; Sánchez Pozo, A.; Rekkas, D.; Volmer, D.; Hirvonen, J.; Bozic, B.; Skowron, A.; Mircioiu, C.; Marcincal, A.; et al. The PHAR-QA project: Competency framework for pharmacy practice—First steps, the results of the European network Delphi round 1. *Pharmacy* **2015**, *3*, 307–329. [CrossRef]
16. Nash, R.E.; Chalmers, L.; Brown, N.; Jackson, S.; Peterson, G. An international review of the use of competency standards in undergraduate pharmacy education. *Pharm. Educ.* **2015**, *15*, 131–141.
17. Plaza, C.M.; Draugalis, J.R.; Slack, M.K.; Skrepnek, G.H.; Sauer, K.A. Curriculum mapping in program assessment and evaluation. *Am. J. Pharm. Educ.* **2007**, *71*, 20. [CrossRef] [PubMed]
18. Atkinson, J.; de Paepe, K.; Sánchez Pozo, A.; Rekkas, D.; Volmer, D.; Hirvonen, J.; Bozic, B.; Skowron, A.; Mircioiu, C.; Marcincal, A.; et al. What is a Pharmacist: Opinions of Pharmacy Department Academics and Community Pharmacists on Competences Required for Pharmacy Practice. *Pharmacy* **2016**, *4*, 12. [CrossRef]
19. Del Castillo Garcia, B. Updates to degrees in pharmacy directed to the professional development for future pharmacists as health specialists. *J. Eur. Assoc. Faculties Pharm.* **2015**. Available online: http://eafponline.eu/wp-content/uploads/2013/04/EPFN_2015_April.pdf (accessed on 27 December 2016).
20. Anderson, L.W.; Krathwohl, D.R.; Airasian, P.W.; Cruikshank, K.A.; Mayer, R.E.; Pintrich, P.R.; Raths, K.; Wittrock, M.C. *A Taxonomy for Learning, Teaching and Assessing: A Revision of Bloom's Taxonomy of Educational Objectives*; Allyn&Bacon: Boston, MA, USA, 2001.
21. Krathwohl, D.R. A revision of Bloom's taxonomy: An overview. *Theory Pract.* **2002**, *41*, 212–218. [CrossRef]
22. Dybekaer, R. Clinical laboratory work: Concept and terms. *Invited opinion. Eur. J. Clin. Chem. Clin. Biochem.* **1997**, *35*, 495–499.
23. Božič, B. Laboratory Medicine as Pharmacists' Competences. In Proceedings of the EAFP Conference 2014, Ljubljana, Slovenia, 22–24 May 2014.
24. Slovene National Higher Education Program 2011–2020, Ministry of Health. Available online: http://www.arhiv.mvzt.gov.si/nc/en/media_room/news/article/101/6960/ (accessed on 28 December 2016).

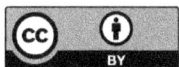

pharmacy

MDPI

Article

Are We Ready to Implement Competence-Based Teaching in Pharmacy Education in Poland?

Agnieszka Skowron *, Justyna Dymek, Anna Gołda and Wioletta Polak

Faculty of Pharmacy, Jagiellonian University Medical College, Krakow 30-699, Poland;
jdymek@cm-uj.krakow.pl (J.D.); annagolda@cm-uj.krakow.pl (A.G.); wpolak@cm-uj.krakow.pl (W.P.)
* Correspondence: agnieszka.skowron@uj.edu.pl; Tel.: +48-12-620-5516

Academic Editor: Jeffrey Atkinson
Received: 4 February 2017; Accepted: 3 May 2017; Published: 9 May 2017

Abstract: Pharmacists in Poland are responsible for the dispensing and quality control of pharmaceuticals. The education process in pharmacy is regulated and monitored at the national level. Pharmacy education at Jagiellonian University is organized in a traditional way based on input and content teaching. The aim of the study was to determinate whether the Jagiellonian University curriculum in the Pharmacy program meets the criteria of the European Competence Framework. The mapping of the *intended curriculum* was done by four academic teachers. The qualitative and quantitative analysis of the distribution of the European Competence Framework among a group of courses and study years was done. We observed that most of the *personal competencies* are offered to students in their senior years, while *the patient care competencies* are distributed equally during the cycle of the study, and only some of them are overrepresented at the senior years. We need a legislation change at the national level as well as organizational and mental change at the university level to move from learning outcome-based pharmacy education to competence-based.

Keywords: learning outcomes; pharmacy; competence framework; higher education institution

1. Introduction

The Pharmacist designation in Poland is recognized in the Polish Health System as a profession responsible for the dispensing and quality control of pharmaceuticals [1]. According to the Constitution of the Republic of Poland, the pharmacist is considered as a "profession in which the public repose confidence, (. . .) and self-governments shall concern themselves with the proper practice of such professions in accordance with, and for the purpose of protecting, the public interest" [2]. It also constitutes pharmacists as a "regulated profession", which is in accordance with the European Directive [3].

The pharmacist profession in Poland is still seen as a stable and well-paid. Analysis of the labor market showed that pharmacy graduates need only about 2–4 weeks to be employed, and during the first two years after graduation, their salaries are higher than any other medical graduates [4]. Due to the European Directive, the Master Diploma in Pharmacy (MDPharm) awarded in Poland is recognized in EU states, which improves the mobility among pharmacists and determines the competitiveness of the profession compared to other graduates [4,5]. Therefore, the main determinant which influenced the decision of young adults in choosing the pharmacy school in Poland is the confidence that in the future they will be able to find a well-paid position in Poland or in EU states [6].

Pharmaceutical education in Poland is based on the Bologna process, which regulation was implemented into the Higher Education System in Poland at the beginning of the XXI century [7,8]. As a regulated profession, the pharmacist is one of the health professions for which education is based on national standards established by law act amended by the Ministry of Science and Higher Education (MSHE) [9].

The National Standards for Pharmacy Education Act consists of five parts: (1) general requirements for pharmacy program, (2) general learning outcomes (gLO), (3) specific learning outcomes (sLO), (4) organization of the process of education, and (5) methods recommended to be used in the assessment process. The minimal requirements for the MDPharm program are the following: 11 semesters with no less than 5300 contact hours at courses and internships and 330 ECTS (European Credit Transfer System) in total. The general and specific learning outcomes are described as learning outcomes in knowledge, professional, and social skills. The specific learning outcomes are grouped into five main dimensions of sciences, such as (A) biomedical and humanistic sciences; (B) physics and chemistry; (C) analysis, synthesis, and technology; (D) biopharmacy and pharmacotherapy outcomes; (E) pharmacy practice; and (F) student's scientific project. In Table 1, the distribution of contact hours and ECTS credits established in the national standard for pharmacy is presented in detail. The learning outcomes in the Polish National Standard for Pharmacy are described separately for knowledge and professional or social skills [9].

Table 1. The National Standard for Pharmacy—distribution of contact hours and credits in the main scientific and internship dimensions [9].

Area	Topic Group Name	Contact Hours for Student (in Total)	ECTS
Basic sciences	(A) biomedical and humanistic sciences	660	98
	(B) physics and chemistry	765	
Pharmaceutical Sciences	(C) analysis, synthesis, and technology	840	140
	(D) biopharmacy and pharmacotherapy outcomes	480	
	(E) pharmacy practice	410	
	(F) scientific project	375	
Internships	(I) holiday internships	320	10
	(IS) senior students internship (6-month)	960	40

Despite the regulation described above, the autonomy of universities empowers academics to develop, plan, and organize the specific MDPharm program as well as to use teaching methods which ensure that student will achieve the learning outcomes established in the national standard [9].

Nowadays, among the ten Faculties of Pharmacy located in the main medical universities in Poland, approximately 1500 students graduate each year, who mainly start their professional work as pharmacists in the community and in hospital pharmacies [4,5]. In the last twenty years in pharmacy education, we observed the tendency to switch from chemistry-based pharmacy which was focused on the medicinal product, to medicine-based pharmacy which is more patient-oriented [10].

Jagiellonian University established a quality control system which aims to analyze and improve the education process to ensure that it fulfills the national standards. The Faculty of Pharmacy at Jagiellonian University Medical College (FP-JUCM) with a 250-year tradition in pharmacy teaching is one of the oldest schools of pharmacy in Central-Eastern Europe and the oldest in Poland; for the last few years, it has also been recognized as the best one in Poland [11].

The education process in the MDPharm at FP-JUCM is organized in a traditional way based on input and content teaching; this means that the student has to participate and pass the final exams of obligatory and optional courses and internships. The course syllabus contains the description of the learning outcomes and information about the teaching and evaluation methods, which are used to ensure that the student will achieve all learning outcomes. The FP-UJCM offers pharmacy students about one hundred separate courses, and half of them are obligatory. Despite obligatory courses, the student is obliged to pass at least twenty-two optional courses. Each of the obligatory courses should cover sLO described in the national standard for pharmacy. In Table 2, detailed information about the distribution of the sLO in the obligatory courses in pharmacy is shown. According to the Polish National Standard for Pharmacy, the MDPharm program covers 5.5 years of courses and internships, including six months of internship in community or hospital pharmacy [9].

Table 2. The quantitative analysis of the distribution of the specific learning outcomes (sLO) into the courses in the Master Diploma in Pharmacy (MDPharm) program at the Faculty of Pharmacy at Jagiellonian University Medical College (FP-JUCM) [9].

Courses in Specific Topic Group	Learning Outcomes (n *)		
	Knowledge	Professional Skills	Social Skills
(A) Biology/Genetics, Anatomy, Physiology, Pathophysiology, Biochemistry, Immunology, Molecular Biology, Microbiology, Botanics, First Aid, Philosophy, Psychology	32	22	3
(B) Biophysics, Inorganic and Organic Chemistry, Analytical Chemistry, Maths, Statistic, IT technology	27	17	3
(C) Medicinal Chemistry, Medicinal synthesis, Biotechnology, Pharmacognosis, Pharmaceutical Technology	41	17	-
(D) Biopharmacy, Pharmacokinetics, Pharmacology, Toxicology, Bromatology, Herbal drugs	47	69	-
(E) Pharmaceutical care, Clinical Pharmacy, Law and Ethics, Pharmacoeconomics, Epidemiology, Drug Information, Pharmacy Practice	55	55	-
(F) Scientific project	2	6	-

* number of learning outcomes in specific category.

A "set of competencies for pharmacists" was presented as one of the results of "Pharmacy Education in Europe—PHARMINE project" Afterwards, The PHAR-QA consortium together with the European Association of Faculties of Pharmacies extended the PHARMINE results to "produce a harmonized model for quality assurance in pharmacy education" [12]. The European Competence Framework (ECF) is one of core results of PHAR-QA project, which could be used in "setting up and/or modifying curricula in European pharmacy departments" [12]. ECF is a list of competencies for pharmacists. They consist of the two major categories—*personal competence* and *patient care competences*, which are divided into four and seven subcategories, respectively [13].

The aim of our study was to determine whether the FP-JUCM curriculum program in the MDPharm meets the criteria of the European Competence Framework [13] and to recognize the gaps and areas which need to be improved if we want our graduates to be a competent and well-educated pharmacist in the future.

2. Materials and Methods

The mapping process was based on "intended curriculum" of the MDPharm program designed and developed at the FP-UJCM. The MDPharm program documents consist of the *courses syllabuses* and the *program matrix table*. The *program matrix table* shows which of the obligatory courses reflect the sLO. The matrix table contains in the horizontal dimension the list of all obligatory courses and in the vertical dimension the list of sLO. The matrix is completed separately every year, and is used in quality control process to ensure that all sLO are presented in MDPharm program content.

The group of four academic teachers from FP-UJCM was involved in the mapping process. All of them were pharmacists who were awarded their Diploma in Pharmacy at Jagiellonian University. Two of the teachers were experienced academics (AS and AG) with at least ten years of experience in research and teaching in pharmaceutical sciences, and two were less-experienced (JD and WP). All teachers worked as community pharmacists in the past. Additionally, one of them (AS) was also employed in the regional office of National Fund of Health, which was a legislative and financial institution.

The mapping process consisted of two steps. In the first step, each academic fulfilled the matrix of competencies (in the vertical dimension) and sLO (in the horizontal dimension). So, the academics had to decide whether the sLO reflects the specific competence (from the European Competence

Framework). In the second step, the matrix of competencies and sLO were translated to courses (from the MDPharm program). We use the *program matrix table* to attribute each competence to a specific obligatory course. A schedule of the mapping process is presented in Figure 1.

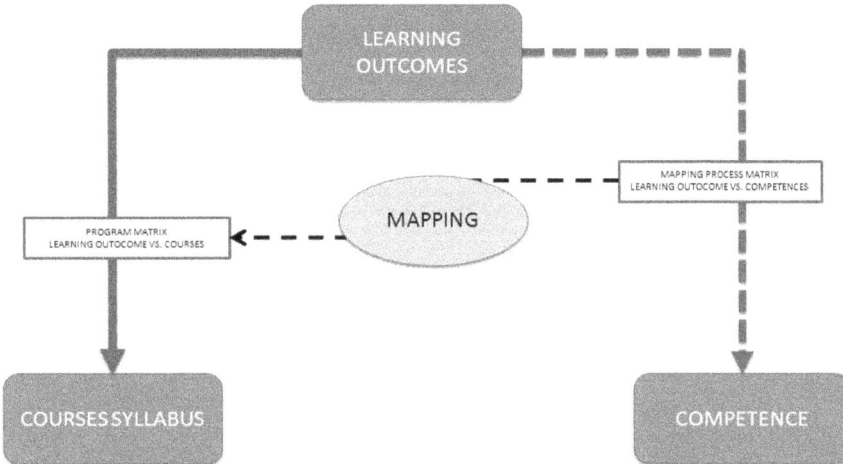

Figure 1. A schedule of the mapping process of the MDPharm program at FP-UJCM.

Finally, a quantitative analysis was done to identify gaps in the existing program. We summarize the number of courses in which learning outcomes in knowledge and skills reflect the specific competence. We also subjectively categorize the required level of the competence using the Dutch Competence Standard Framework, which consists of five levels. The gradation of students' knowledge, skills, and professional behavior starts from level one, where the student demonstrates knowledge and basic professional behavior and ends on level five, where student "independently performs the professional activity" [14].

3. Results

3.1. Matrix of Learning Outcomes versus Competence

We assumed that a specific competence was reflected by a specific learning outcome if it was marked by at least two of the academics. The qualitative analysis of the competence vs. learning outcomes matrix showed the following:

- each competence was reflected by 23 sLO on average (the median value = 20), the maximum number of sLO reflecting the separate competence was 72, and there were two competencies which was not reflected by any of sLO; on average, competencies were reflected by 13 knowledge sLO (the median value = 10) and 10 skills sLO (the median value = 9)
- each sLO reflected three competencies on average (the median value = 2), most sLO reflected two competencies (mode)

The detailed data of some knowledge and skills sLO covering the group of competencies is presented in Table 3.

Table 3. Qualitative and quantitative analysis of the distribution of the learning outcomes in the European Competence Framework (ECF) [9,12].

		Learning outcomes	
		Knowledge	Skills
1. Personal competences: learning and knowledge	1.1. Ability to identify learning needs and to learn independently (including continuous professional development (CPD)).	1	1
	1.2. Ability to apply logic to problem solving.	0	0
	1.3. Ability to critically appraise relevant knowledge and to summarise the key points.	1	1
	1.4. Ability to evaluate scientific data in line with current scientific and technological knowledge.	3	12
	1.5. Ability to apply preclinical and clinical evidence-based medical science to pharmaceutical practice.	10	14
	1.6. Ability to apply current knowledge of relevant legislation and codes of pharmacy practice.	15	9
2. Personal competences: values	2.1. A professional approach to tasks and human relations.	3	2
	2.2. Ability to maintain confidentiality.	4	2
	2.3. Ability to take full responsibility for patient care.	7	1
	2.4. Ability to inspire the confidence of others in one's actions and advice.	8	1
	2.5. Knowledge of appropriate legislation and of ethics.	24	10
3. Personal competences: communication and organisational skills.	3.1. Ability to communicate effectively—both oral and written—in the locally relevant language.	2	4
	3.2. Ability to effectively use information technology.	3	7
	3.3. Ability to work effectively as part of a team.	5	6
	3.4. Ability to implement general legal requirements that impact upon the practice of pharmacy (e.g., health and safety legislation, employment law).	8	1
	3.5. Ability to contribute to the training of staff.	4	1
	3.6. Ability to manage risk and quality of service issues.	1	1
	3.7. Ability to identify the need for new services.	0	0
	3.8. Ability to understand a business environment and develop entrepreneurship.	2	1
4. Personal competences: research and industrial pharmacy.	4.1. Knowledge of design, synthesis, isolation, characterisation and biological evaluation of active substances.	56	15
	4.2. Knowledge of good manufacturing practice and of good laboratory practice.	29	34
	4.3. Knowledge of European directives on qualified persons.	3	3
	4.4. Knowledge of drug registration, licensing and marketing.	11	9
	4.5. Knowledge of the importance of research in pharmaceutical development and practice.	24	16
5. Patient care competences—patient consultation and assessment.	5.1. Ability to interpret basic medical laboratory tests.	6	13
	5.2. Ability to perform appropriate diagnostic tests e.g., measurement of blood pressure or blood sugar.	4	7
	5.3. Ability to recognise when referral to another member of the healthcare team is needed.	8	0
6. Patient care competences—need for drug treatment.	6.1. Ability to retrieve and interpret information on the patient's clinical background.	25	2
	6.2. Ability to compile and interpret a comprehensive drug history for an individual patient.	5	2
	6.3. Ability to identify non-adherence to medicine therapy and make an appropriate intervention.	3	0
	6.4. Ability to advise physicians on the appropriateness of prescribed medicines and—in some cases—to prescribe medication.	17	23

Table 3. *Cont.*

		Learning outcomes	
		Knowledge	Skills
7. Patient care competences–drug interactions.	7.1. Ability to identify and prioritise drug-drug interactions and advise appropriate changes to medication.	23	14
	7.2. Ability to identify and prioritise drug-patient interactions, including those that prevent or require the use of a specific drug, based on pharmaco-genetics, and advise on appropriate changes to medication.	29	13
	7.3. Ability to identify and prioritise drug-disease interactions (e.g., NSAIDs in heart failure) and advise on appropriate changes to medication.	11	14
8. Patient care competences: drug dose and formulation.	8.1. Knowledge of the bio-pharmaceutical, pharmacodynamic and pharmacokinetic activity of a substance in the body.	42	30
	8.2. Ability to recommend interchangeability of drugs based on in-depth understanding and knowledge of bioequivalence, bio-similarity and therapeutic equivalence of drugs.	24	21
	8.3. Ability to undertake a critical evaluation of a prescription ensuring that it is clinically appropriate and legally valid.	15	5
	8.4. Knowledge of the supply chain of medicines thus ensuring timely flow of quality drug products to the patient.	3	0
	8.5. Ability to manufacture medicinal products that are not commercially available.	17	7
9. Patient care competences–patient education.	9.1. Ability to promote public health in collaboration with other professionals within the healthcare system.	9	9
	9.2. Ability to provide appropriate lifestyle advice to improve patient outcomes (e.g., advice on smoking, obesity, etc.).	24	12
	9.3. Ability to use pharmaceutical knowledge and provide evidence-based advice on public health issues involving medicines.	30	8
10. Patient care competences–provision of information and service.	10.1. Ability to use effective consultations to identify the patient's need for information.	18	9
	10.2. Ability to provide accurate and appropriate information on prescription medicines.	22	34
	10.3. Ability to provide evidence-based support for patients in selection and use of non-prescription medicines.	24	30
11. Patient care competences–monitoring of drug therapy.	11.1. Ability to identify and prioritise problems in the management of medicines in a timely and effective manner and so ensure patient safety.	12	22
	11.2. Ability to monitor and report Adverse Drug Events and Adverse Drug Reactions (ADEs and ADRs) to all concerned, in a timely manner, and in accordance with current regulatory guidelines on Good Pharmacovigilance Practices (GVPs).	21	17
	11.3. Ability to undertake a critical evaluation of prescribed medicines to confirm that current clinical guidelines are appropriately applied.	19	14
	11.4. Ability to monitor patient care outcomes to optimise treatment in collaboration with the prescriber.	18	20
	11.5. Ability to contribute to the cost effectiveness of treatment by collection and analysis of data on medicines use.	10	19

3.2. Matrix of Competencies versus Courses

The courses were grouped according to the scientific fields (as described in Table 3) and to the year of the study; we also included the scientific project, holiday, and final internships.

Most of the *Personal competencies in learning and knowledge* are covered by the courses in group C, which are offered mostly at final years of the study. The *Personal competencies: Values* are covered by the first and senior years of study, which offer ethics courses on the one hand, and on the other the senior internship, where the student has an opportunity to observe "real life" and to develop their attitude toward the ethical dilemma. The *Personal competencies such as communication and organization skills and research and industrial pharmacy* seem to be balanced between all groups of courses and all study years. The details of the distribution of *personal competencies* between topic groups and the years of the MDPharm are shown in Table 4.

The *Patient Care Competencies* are less covered by courses from the group B (physics and chemistry), which are mainly offered to the second year students. FP-UJCM students may achieve most of the *Patient Care Competencies* at the senior years of their MDPharm (fourth to sixth years). The details of the distribution of *Patient Care Competencies* between topic groups and years of the MDPharm are shown in Table 5.

Table 4. Quantitative analysis of the distribution of the *Personal competencies* into the group of courses or the study year at FP-UJ CM [12].

	PERSONAL COMPETENCE	GROUP A (n = 13)	GROUP B (n = 8)	GROUP A (n = 13)	GROUP D (N = 6)	GROUP E (N = 10)	YEAR 1 (N = 13)	YEAR 2 (N = 6)	YEAR 3 (N = 8)	YEAR 4 (N = 10)	YEAR 5+6 (N = 9)
		n	n	n	n	n	n	n	n	n	n
LEARNING AND KNOWLEDGE	1.1. Ability to identify learning needs and to learn independently (including continuous professional development (CPD)).						1				1
	1.2. Ability to apply logic to problem solving.										
	1.3. Ability to critically appraise relevant knowledge and to summarise the key points.						1			1	1
	1.4. Ability to evaluate scientific data in line with current scientific and technological knowledge.	4	1				4	4	1	2	2
	1.5. Ability to apply preclinical and clinical evidence-based medical science to pharmaceutical practice.		1			3	5	1		4	4
	1.6. Ability to apply current knowledge of relevant legislation and codes of pharmacy practice.	1					7	1		2	5
VALUES	2.1. A professional approach to tasks and human relations.	3					4	1	1	1	4
	2.2. Ability to maintain confidentiality.	2				1	2	1	1	1	2
	2.3. Ability to take full responsibility for patient care.	1					3		1		3
	2.4. Ability to inspire the confidence of others in one's actions and advice.	2					5	1	1		5
	2.5. Knowledge of appropriate legislation and of ethics.	1				1	6	1		2	5
COMMUNICATION AND ORGANISATIONAL SKILLS	3.1. Ability to communicate effectively–both oral and written–in the locally relevant language.	1	2	1	2	2	2		2	2	2
	3.2. Ability to effectively use information technology.		4				2	3	1		2
	3.3. Ability to work effectively as part of a team.	1	3		1		3	2	1	2	2
	3.4. Ability to implement general legal requirements that impact upon the practice of pharmacy (e.g., health and safety legislation, employment law).						4				4
	3.5. Ability to contribute to the training of staff.	3						1	1	1	
	3.6. Ability to manage risk and quality of service issues.	1		2				1		1	1
	3.7. Ability to identify the need for new services.										
	3.8. Ability to understand a business environment and develop entrepreneurship.						1				1
RESEARCH AND INDUSTRIAL PHARMACY	4.1. Knowledge of design, synthesis, isolation, characterisation and biological evaluation of active substances.	2	7	5	4		5	4	2	3	3
	4.2. Knowledge of good manufacturing practice and of good laboratory practice.	8	3	7	4		5	4	5	4	3
	4.3. Knowledge of European directives on qualified persons.			4	2				2	1	2
	4.4. Knowledge of drug registration, licensing and marketing.			6	1	7			2	3	8
	4.5. Knowledge of the importance of research in pharmaceutical development and practice.	1	4	7	2	1	4	1	2	4	3

N–total number of courses in the group or study year, n–number of courses reflecting the specific competence.

Table 5. Quantitative analysis of the distribution of the *Patient care competencies* into the topic groups or the year of the pharmacy course at FP-UJ CM [12].

	PATIENT CARE COMPETENCE	GROUP A (n = 13)	GROUP B (n = 8)	GROUP C (n = 13)	GROUP D (N = 6)	GROUP E (N = 10)	YEAR 1 (N = 13)	YEAR 2 (N = 6)	YEAR 3 (N = 8)	YEAR 4 (N = 10)	YEAR 5+6 (N = 9)
		n	n	n	n	n	n	n	n	n	n
PATIENT CONSULTATION AND ASSESSMENT	5.1. Ability to interpret basic medical laboratory tests.	5	1	1			1	2	2	3	1
	5.2. Ability to perform appropriate diagnostic tests e.g., measurement of blood pressure or blood sugar.	4	1	1				2	2	2	
	5.3. Ability to recognize when referral to another member of the healthcare team is needed.	1			2	4			1	2	4
NEED FOR DRUG TREATMENT	6.1. Ability to retrieve and interpret information on the patient's clinical background.	9		2		2	3	3	3	1	2
	6.2. Ability to compile and interpret a comprehensive drug history for an individual patient.	1		1	1	2			1	2	2
	6.3. Ability to identify non-adherence to medicine therapy and make an appropriate intervention.					2					2
	6.4. Ability to advise physicians on the appropriateness of prescribed medicines and–in some cases–to prescribe medication.	1	1	5	5	6	1		3	5	8
DRUG INTERACTIONS	7.1. Ability to identify and prioritise drug-drug interactions and advise appropriate changes to medication.	7		1	5	2	3	2	4	3	3
	7.2. Ability to identify and prioritise drug-patient interactions, including those that prevent or require the use of a specific drug, based on pharmaco-genetics, and advise on appropriate changes to medication.	6		3	5	2	2	2	4	3	4
	7.3. Ability to identify and prioritise drug-disease interactions (e.g., NSAIDs in heart failure) and advise on appropriate changes to medication.			3	5	2			2	3	4
DRUG DOSE AND FORMULATION	8.1. Knowledge of the bio-pharmaceutical, pharmacodynamic and pharmacokinetic activity of a substance in the body.	9	1	6	5	2	4	3	6	5	4
	8.2. Ability to recommend interchangeability of drugs based on in-depth understanding and knowledge of bioequivalence, bio-similarity and therapeutic equivalence of drugs.			6	6				3	5	3
	8.3. Ability to undertake a critical evaluation of a prescription ensuring that it is clinically appropriate and legally valid.			5	4	2			3	3	4
	8.4. Knowledge of the supply chain of medicines thus ensuring timely flow of quality drug products to the patient.					2					2
	8.5. Ability to manufacture medicinal products that are not commercially available.	1		5	3	1	1		3	2	3
PATIENT EDUCATION	9.1. Ability to promote public health in collaboration with other professionals within the healthcare system.	4			2	2		1	3	1	3
	9.2. Ability to provide appropriate lifestyle advice to improve patient outcomes (e.g., advice on smoking, obesity, etc.).	9			2	1	3	3	3	2	1
	9.3. Ability to use pharmaceutical knowledge and provide evidence-based advice on public health issues involving medicines.	6			3	4	2	2	2	4	3
PROVISION OF INFORMATION AND SERVICE	10.1. Ability to use effective consultations to identify the patient's need for information.	5			2	5	3		2	3	4
	10.2. Ability to provide accurate and appropriate information on prescription medicines.	2		5	5	5	1		3	5	7
	10.3. Ability to provide evidence-based support for patients in selection and use of non-prescription medicines.	2		5	5	5	1		3	4	8
MONITORING OF DRUG THERAPY	11.1. Ability to identify and prioritise problems in the management of medicines in a timely and effective manner and so ensure patient safety.	1		3	4	4	1		2	3	6
	11.2. Ability to monitor and report Adverse Drug Events and Adverse Drug Reactions (ADEs and ADRs) to all concerned, in a timely manner, and in accordance with current regulatory guidelines on Good Pharmacovigilance Practices (GVPs).				4	4	4		1	6	5
	11.3. Ability to undertake a critical evaluation of prescribed medicines to confirm that current clinical guidelines are appropriately applied.	2		5	6	7	2		3	7	8
	11.4. Ability to monitor patient care outcomes to optimize treatment in collaboration with the prescriber.	1	1	5	5	6	2		2	6	8
	11.5. Ability to contribute to the cost effectiveness of treatment by collection and analysis of data on medicines use.	4	4	2	4	3	1		2	4	4

N–total number of courses in the group or study year, n–number of courses reflecting the specific competence.

3.3. Analysis of the Level of Competencies

We based our subjective analysis (which reflects the levels of the *Dutch Competence Standard Framework*) on the document on the one hand, and our personal experience as a pharmacist and a teacher on the other. Two of our colleagues (JD and WP) could also use their experience as a pharmacy student because at least half of their courses were established basing on Bologna process. We also took into account the composition of knowledge sLO and skills sLO covering the specific competence as well as a teaching and assessing methods described in the course syllabus. The results of our discussion are presented in Table 6. In the brackets, we listed the numbers of the competencies (according to the Tables 4 and 5) which could be achieved on the specific level at the end of the MDPharm program.

Table 6. A desk analysis of the level of competence achieved by a student at the MDPharm program at FP-UJCM [14].

		Level *
Personal Competencies	learning and knowledge	1a (1,3,4); 1c (5,6)
	values	2 (3,4); 3 (5); 4 (1,2)
	communication and organisational skills	1a (1,3); 1c (4); 2 (6); 3 (7,8); 4 (2)
	research and industrial pharmacy	1c (3,5); 3 (2,4); 5 (1)
Patient Care Competencies	patient consultation and assessment	1a (1,3)
	need for drug treatment	1a (2,3); 1c (1,4)
	drug interactions	1a (1); 2 (2,3)
	drug dose and formulation	1c (2); 2 (5); 3 (1,4); 4 (3)
	patient education	1c (2); 2 (3); 3 (1)
	provision of information and service	1c (1); 2 (2,3)
	monitoring of drug therapy	1a (3,5); 2 (1); 4 (2,4)

* the level of Dutch Competence Standard Framework; in the brackets, we used the numbers of the specific competencies from Tables 4 and 5.

Most of the competencies (n = 12) seem to be possible to be achieved by students on the level 1 (1a to 1 c), which is a basic level and means that a student can present the knowledge and demonstrate professional behavior only in a test situation.

4. Discussion

The mapping process of the curriculum at the FP-UJCM was a part of the cooperation of the partners of the PHAR-QA Consortium [12], and by the discussion between partners, it was limited to "intended curriculum" mapping. We mapped the "intended curriculum" based only on official documents of the MDPharm program at our faculty, which means that the results of our analysis did not reflect the opinion of the students or another teacher. We hope it can be used to identify the gaps and to see what could be improved in future [15].

The MDPharm program at Jagiellonian University is based on learning outcomes defined at the national level [9]. It educates students to be future professional staff in a community and hospital pharmacy, so the patient-oriented European Competence Framework [13] should be widely represented and recognized in the curriculum documents.

In the first step of our analysis, we had to "translate" the sLO created for knowledge, professional, and social skills into the competencies. We observed a high inconsistency among the total number of sLO, which could be recognized as reflecting the specific *Personal competencies*. For example, we found:

– 71 sLO (56 in knowledge and 15 in skills) which we matched to competence: *Knowledge of design, synthesis, isolation, characterization and biological evaluation of active substances* (4.1 in Table 3)
– only two sLO (one in knowledge and one in skills) for competencies:

  ○ *ability to identify learning needs and to learn independently (including continuous professional development (CPD)-1.1 in Table 3);*

    ○   *ability to critically appraise relevant knowledge and to summarize the key points (1.3 in Table 3);*
    ○   *ability to manage risk and quality of service issues (see 3.6 in Table 3).*

−   two Personal competence: *ability to apply logic to problem-solving* (1.2 in Table 3) and *ability to identify the need for new services* (3.7 in Table 3), which we could not recognize as directly represented by sLO, and consequently, delivered by any obligatory course.

A similar situation was recognized in the group of *Patient care competencies*, where:

−   72 sLO (42 in knowledge and 30 in skills) reflected the competence *Knowledge of the bio-pharmaceutical, pharmacodynamic and pharmacokinetic activity of a substance in the body* (8.1 in Table 3)

−   only three sLO (in knowledge) reflected the competence *Ability to identify non-adherence to medicine therapy and make an appropriate intervention* (6.3 in Table 3) and *Knowledge of the supply chain of medicines thus ensuring timely flow of quality drug products to the patient* (8.4 in Table 3).

The analysis of the distribution of competences among the study years (Tables 4 and 5) showed that a student has an opportunity to achieve *personal competencies* mostly during the senior years of the study (5th and 6th year). Only competencies in *research and industrial pharmacy* are distributed equally at the junior and senior years of the study. Students achieve the *patient care competencies* at the 3rd, 4th, 5th, and 6th years of the study. However, most of them—especially in the group *provision of information and services*—are distributed among the courses of the last three years (4th to 6th).

Based on the Dutch Competence Standard Framework [14], we also tried to subjectively assess the level of competencies achieved by the student [14]. In general, we assumed (Table 6) that most competencies are achieved at a level 1 or 2. There is a limited group of competencies among *Personal competencies* and *patient care competencies* which could be considered as achieved at the 4th level, and only one—*knowledge of design, synthesis, isolation, characterization and biological evaluation of active substances*—which could be achieved at a level 5. We can conclude that despite wide reflection of the *need for drug treatment* or *provision of information and service* competencies in the sLO, the subjective assessment showed that it is highly possible that a student can only present the knowledge about the specific competence and demonstrate the skills only in a test situation. This means that she is not "able to adequately carry out professional activities in an authentic professional situation under the supervision of an experienced practitioner" [14].

A major limitation of the mapping process based on "intended curriculum" is the fact that it is based on documents only, so we could not be sure that the ideas described in documents are implemented into the daily teaching activity. This means that even those competencies which we recognized as "well" reflected by the sLO might not be achieved by all students. To verify the results of our study, we plan to extend the analysis, and we are planning the study of the student's perception about their competencies.

Because the results of our analysis already showed gaps and lack of balance between competencies and learning outcomes, we will recommend Dean's office to start the discussion with the teachers at FP-UJ CM to encourage them to switch to competence-based learning.

The main conclusion of our analysis is that the education system for pharmacy in Poland based on learning outcomes does not directly reflect the competencies. This means that to start with competence-based pharmacy education, we need to change the legal regulation at the national level and redefine our teaching at the university level. Despite the changes in the national regulations in the pharmacy field, academics should remember that their main obligation is to ensure that their graduates will be able to work independently and responsibly to improve the health of the society and to ensure the safe and effective use of drugs. As academics who are experienced in teaching, we have to be aware of our responsibility for creating the professional attitude and competencies of our students. As pharmacists and academics, we are also responsible for developing the professional education system to let our students become the professionals of the future.

Author Contributions: A.S. conceived and designed the experiments; A.S., J.D., A.G., and W.P prepared the tools and performed the mapping process; A.S. analyzed the data and wrote the paper.

Conflicts of Interest: The authors declare no conflict of interest.

References

1. The Pharmaceutical Law of 6th September 2001. Available online: http://isap.sejm.gov.pl/DetailsServlet?id=WDU20011261381 (accessed on 7 January 2017). (In Polish)
2. The Constitution of The Republic of Poland of 2nd April 1997 as published in Dziennik Ustaw No. 78, item 483. Available online: http://www.sejm.gov.pl/prawo/konst/angielski/konse.htm (accessed on 10 January 2017).
3. Directive 2005/36/EC of the European Parliament and of the Council of 7th September 2005 on the recognition of professional qualifications. *Off. J. Eur. Union* **2005**, *48*, 22–142. Available online: http://eur-lex.europa.eu/legal-content/EN/TXT/?uri=OJ:L:2005:255:TOC (accessed on 20 January 2017).
4. The Professional Career of the Graduates of the Faculty of Pharmacy of the Jagiellonian University Medical College in the academic year 2014/2015—Report. Available online: http://www.sdka.cm.uj.edu.pl/documents/13606729/32429686/Raport%20losy%20absolwent%C3%B3w%20-%20Wydzia%C5%82%20Farmaceutyczny%2014_15.pdf (accessed on 10 January 2017). (In Polish)
5. Report on economic aspects of the career of the graduates of the Faculty of Pharmacy of the Jagiellonian University Medical College. Available online: http://absolwenci.nauka.gov.pl/reports/UJK_6446.pdf (accessed on 23 January 2017).
6. Schulz, A. Motivation for Pursuing a Career in Pharmacy. In *Economic Notes. Selected Economic and Social Problems within the Economies of Poland and the World*; Grzywacz, J., Kowalski, S., Eds.; PWSZ: Płock, Poland, 2014; Volume 20, pp. 135–143. Available online: http://www.wydawnictwo.pwszplock.pl/Ekonomia/nauki_ekonomiczne_20.pdf (accessed on 10 January 2017).
7. Law Act of 27th July 2005 on Higher Education Law as published in Dziennik Ustaw 2016, item 1842. Available online: http://isap.sejm.gov.pl/DetailsServlet?id=WDU20160001842 (accessed on 10 January 2017).
8. Joint declaration of the European Ministers of Education—The Bologna Declaration of 19 June 1999. Available online: http://www.ehea.info/cid100210/ministerial-conference-bologna-1999.html (accessed on 23 January 2017).
9. Regulation of the Minister of Science and Higher Education of 9th May 2012 on education standards for fields of study: Medicine, dentistry, pharmacy, nursing and midwifery as published in Dziennik Ustaw 2012, item 631. Available online: http://isap.sejm.gov.pl/DetailsServlet?id=WDU20120000631 (accessed on 8 January 2017).
10. Atkinson, J. Heterogeneity of Pharmacy Education in Europe. *Pharmacy* **2014**, *2*, 231–243. [CrossRef]
11. Ranking of the Faculties of Pharmacy in Poland in the year 2016. Available online: http://www.perspektywy.pl/RSW2016/ranking-kierunkow-studiow/kierunki-medyczne-i-o-zdrowiu/farmacja (accessed on 20 January 2017).
12. Atkinson, J.; Rombaut, B.; Sánchez Pozo, A.; Rekkas, D.; Veeski, P.; Hirvonen, J.; Bozic, B.; Skowron, A.; Mircioiu, C. A description of the European Pharmacy Education and Training Quality Assurance Project. *Pharmacy* **2013**, *1*, 3–7. [CrossRef]
13. Atkinson, J.; de Paepe, K.; Sánchez Pozo, A.; Rekkas, D.; Volmer, D.; Hirvonen, J.; Bozic, B.; Skowron, A.; Mircioiu, C.; Marcincal, A.; et al. The PHAR-QA project: Competency framework for pharmacy practice—First steps, the results of the European network Delphi round 1. *Pharmacy* **2015**, *3*, 307–329. [CrossRef]
14. 2016 Pharmacist Competency Framework and Domain-Specific Frame of Reference for Netherlands. Available online: https://www.knmp.nl/downloads/pharmacist-competency-frameworkandDSFR-Netherlands.pdf (accessed on 20 January 2017).
15. Kelley, K.A.; Demb, A. Instrumentation for Comparing Student and Faculty Perceptions of Competency-based Assessment. *Am. J. Pharm. Educ.* **2006**, *70*, 134. [CrossRef] [PubMed]

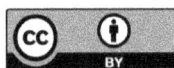

MDPI AG

St. Alban-Anlage 66

4052 Basel, Switzerland

Tel. +41 61 683 77 34

Fax +41 61 302 89 18

http://www.mdpi.com

Pharmacy Editorial Office

E-mail: pharmacy@mdpi.com

http://www.mdpi.com/journal/pharmacy

www.ingramcontent.com/pod-product-compliance
Lightning Source LLC
Chambersburg PA
CBHW051904210326

41597CB00033B/6020